HISTOLOGICAL TYPING OF SKIN TUMOURS

⌐HISTOLOGICAL TYPING
OF SKIN TUMOURS

R. E. J. ᴛᴇɴ SELDAM

*Head, WHO International Reference Centre
for the Histological Classification
of Skin Tumours, Department of Pathology,
School of Medicine,
University of Western Australia,
Perth, Australia*

E. B. HELWIG

*Pathologist,
Armed Forces Institute of Pathology,
Washington D.C., USA*

in collaboration with

L. H. SOBIN

*Pathologist, Cancer,
World Health Organization,
Geneva, Switzerland*

H. TORLONI

*Medical Officer, Research and Development,
Pan American Health Organization,
Washington, D.C., USA*

and pathologists in eleven countries

WORLD HEALTH ORGANIZATION

GENEVA

1974

LIST OF CENTRES AND REVIEWERS

WHO International Reference Centre for the Histological Classification of Skin Tumours

Head of Centre

DR R. E. J. ten SELDAM, Department of Pathology, School of Medicine, University of Western Australia, Perth, Australia

Collaborating Centres

DR J. CIVATTE, Hôpital Saint-Louis, Paris, France
DR E. B. HELWIG, Armed Forces Institute of Pathology, Washington D.C., USA
DR J. MICHALANY, Department of Pathology, Escola Paulista de Medicina, São Paulo, Brazil
DR L. A. M. MUSSO, Kanematsu Institute of Pathology, Sydney Hospital, Sydney, Australia
DR W. SANDRITTER, Institute of Pathology of the Albert-Ludwig University, Freiburg-in-Breisgau, Federal Republic of Germany
DR SHU YEH, Taiwan University, Taipei, Taiwan
DR E. WEISS, Institute of Veterinary Pathology of the Justus Liebig University, Giessen, Federal Republic of Germany

Reviewers

DR A. POIARES BAPTISTA, Clinic of Dermatology and Venereology, University Hospital of Coimbra, Portugal
DR A. BOURLOND, Clinic of Dermatology, Hôpital St.-Pierre, Louvain, Belgium
DR R. E. KAVETSKY, Institute for Oncological Problems, Kiev, USSR
DR F. KERDEL-VEGAS, Central University of Venezuela and Vargas Hospital, Caracas, Venezuela
DR WANDA NIEPOLOMSKA, Institute of Oncology, Department of Tumour Biology, Gliwice, Poland
DR K. SANDERSON, St George's Hospital, London, England

The photomicrographs reproduced in this volume were taken by Mr H. Upeniek, Department of Pathology, University of Western Australia, Perth, Australia, and Mr C. Edwards, Armed Forces Institute of Pathology, Washington D.C., USA

CONTENTS

Colour photomicrographs

GENERAL PREFACE TO THE SERIES

Among the prerequisites for comparative studies of cancer are international agreement on histological criteria for the classification of cancer types and a standardized nomenclature. At present, pathologists use different terms for the same pathological entity, and furthermore the same term is sometimes applied to lesions of different types. An internationally agreed classification of tumours, acceptable alike to physicians, surgeons, radiologists, pathologists and statisticians, would enable cancer workers in all parts of the world to compare their findings and would facilitate collaboration among them.

In a report published in 1952,[1] a subcommittee of the WHO Expert Committee on Health Statistics discussed the general principles that should govern the statistical classification of tumours and agreed that, to ensure the necessary flexibility and ease in coding, three separate classifications were needed according to (1) anatomical site, (2) histological type, and (3) degree of malignancy. A classification according to anatomical site is available in the International Classification of Diseases.[2]

The question of establishing a universally accepted classification by histological type has received much attention during the last 20 years and a particularly valuable Atlas of Tumor Pathology—*already numbering more than 40 volumes—is being published in the USA by the Armed Forces Institute of Pathology under the auspices of the National Research Council. An* Illustrated Tumour Nomenclature *in English, French, German, Latin, Russian, and Spanish has also been published by the International Union Against Cancer (UICC).*

In 1956 the WHO Executive Board passed a resolution[3] requesting the Director-General to explore the possibility that WHO might organize centres in various parts of the world and arrange for the collection of human tissues and their histological classification. The main purpose of such centres would be to develop histological definitions of cancer types and to facilitate the wide adoption of a uniform nomenclature. This resolution was endorsed by the Tenth World Health Assembly in May 1957[4] and the following month a Study Group on Histological Classification of Cancer Types met in Oslo to advise WHO on its implementation. The Group recommended criteria for selecting tumour sites for study and suggested a procedure for the drafting

[1] *Wld Hlth Org. techn. Rep., Ser.*, 1952, No. 53, p. 45.
[3] World Health Organization (1967) *Manual of the International Statistical Classification of Diseases, Injuries, and Causes of Death*, 1965 revision, Geneva.
[3] *Off. Rec. Wld Hlth Org.*, 1956, **68**, 14 (Resolution EB17.R40).
[4] *Off. Rec. Wld Hlth Org.*, 1957, **79**, 467 (Resolution WHA10.18).

of histological classifications and testing their validity. Briefly, the procedure is as follows:

For each tumour site, a tentative histopathological typing and classification is drawn up by a group of experts, consisting of up to ten pathologists working in the field in question. An international reference centre and a number of collaborating laboratories are then designated by WHO to evaluate the proposed classification. These laboratories exchange histological preparations, accompanied by clinical information. The histological typing is then made in accordance with the proposed classification. Subsequently, one or more technical meetings are called by WHO to facilitate an exchange of opinions and the classification is amended to take account of criticisms.

In addition to preparing the publication and the photomicrographs for it, the reference centre produces up to 100 sets of microscope slides showing the major histological types for distribution to national societies of pathology.

Since 1958, WHO has established 23 international reference centres covering tumours of the lung; breast; soft tissues; oropharynx; bone; ovaries; salivary glands; thyroid; skin; male urogenital tract; jaws; uterus; stomach and oesophagus; intestines; central nervous system; liver, biliary tract and pancreas; upper respiratory tract; eye; and endocrine glands; as well as oral precancerous conditions; the leukaemias and lymphomas; comparative oncology; and exfoliative cytology. This work has involved more than 250 pathologists from over 50 countries. The international reference centres for tumours of the lung; breast; soft tissues; oropharynx; bone; jaws; salivary glands; skin; ovaries; urinary bladder; testis; female genital tract; and intestines; and for leukaemias and lymphomas have completed their work, and most of the classifications prepared by these centres have already been published (see page 6).

The World Health Organization is indebted to the many pathologists who have participated and are participating in this large undertaking, especially to the heads of the international reference centres and of the collaborating laboratories. The pioneer work of many other international and national organizations in the field of histological classification of tumours has greatly facilitated the task undertaken by WHO. Particular gratitude is expressed to the National Cancer Institute, USA, which, through the National Research Council, is providing financial support to accelerate this work Finally, WHO wishes to record its appreciation of the valuable help it has received from the International Council of Societies of Pathology (ICSP) in proposing collaborating centres and in undertaking to distribute copies of the classifications, with corresponding sets of microscope slides, to national societies of pathology all over the world.

PREFACE TO HISTOLOGICAL TYPING
OF SKIN TUMOURS

The WHO International Reference Centre for the Histological Classification of Skin Tumours was established in 1965 at the Department of Pathology, School of Medicine, University of Western Australia, Perth, Australia.

The Centre distributed histological sections from selected cases to the collaborating centres, a list of which will be found on page 5, for typing according to a tentative classification drawn up at a WHO meeting in 1965. In all, 397 cases were studied by these centres and were reviewed at meetings in 1968 and 1970 attended by the heads of the centres. The classification and the definitions and nomenclature used were amended at these meetings in the light of the comments received. After further review by pathologists designated by WHO, the final version of the classification was adopted. The authors then prepared the accompanying text and illustrations.

Most of the colour photomicrographs appearing in this book are also available as a collection of transparencies intended especially for teaching purposes. To help those who might wish to know the corresponding terms in French, Russian, and Spanish, translations of the classification into these languages are also given, immediately following the English version.

It will, of course, be appreciated that the classification reflects the present state of knowledge and that modifications are almost certain to be needed as experience accumulates. Although the present classification has been adopted by the members of the group, it necessarily represents a majority view from which some pathologists may wish to dissent. It is nevertheless hoped that in the interests of international cooperation, all pathologists will try to use the classification as put forward. Criticisms and suggestions for its improvement will be welcomed.

The publications in the series International Histological Classification of Tumours *are not intended to serve as textbooks but rather to promote the adoption of a uniform terminology and categorization of tumours that will facilitate and improve communication among cancer workers. For this reason the literature references in general have intentionally been kept to a minimum; in this particular volume no references are given as the number of lesions and conditions covered by the classification would need far too extensive a bibliography.*

INTRODUCTION

In a classification of tumours, it is necessary to define what is meant by the word " tumour ". In the classical sense, " tumour " simply means a swelling, but nowadays it is customary to use the term to mean a new growth or neoplasm. It is in this sense that the term is used in this classification. Even so, it must be remembered that practically any pathological condition affecting the skin, be it degenerative, inflammatory, vascular, metabolic, or neoplastic in nature, can lead to a swelling, and that it commonly does so. In these cases, it is sometimes extremely difficult to decide clinically, and occasionally also histologically, whether the swelling is a real neoplasm or a pseudotumour. Consequently, it is not surprising that different authors hold different views as to the exact classification of skin tumours.

The skin is the largest organ of the body. In addition, it is complex in its structure and varies from one part of the body to another. Epidermis, hair follicles, sweat glands, sebaceous glands, the soft tissue components of the corium, and even the subcutis can all be involved in tumour formations that are either characteristically cutaneous in character or more common in the skin than elsewhere in the body. Some of these lesions are a cutaneous expression of tumours elsewhere in the body or are part of a systemic disease.

It is customary to divide tumours into malignant and benign categories, but it must be remembered that biological processes are usually continuous and that a sharp division between " malignant " and " benign " does not always exist. For instance, basal cell carcinoma is a relatively benign lesion and generally speaking easily cured. This has resulted in the introduction of other terms to avoid the use of " carcinoma ", but we believe that a lesion that extends relentlessly when not actively interfered with and that does occasionally kill is best classified as a carcinoma. Dermatofibrosarcoma protuberans is not as malignant as the name indicates but it has a tendency to persistent recurrences and for that reason is better classified among the malignant tumours. The exact nature of a number of lesions is in doubt and some of them may well be malformations or hamartomas. It would be wrong, however, in the present state of knowledge, to make too many divisions that are based only on assumptions and not on scientific evidence.

Terminology and principles of classification

This classification lists those tumours and pseudotumours that arise in any part of the cutis or that involve this organ in a more or less characteristic way. Where appropriate, reference is made in the explanatory notes to other classifications of tumours published by WHO, particularly to *Histological Typing of Soft Tissue Tumours* (No. 3 in this series, see p. 6), which complements the present classification in many respects.

One of the difficulties encountered in drawing up the classification was what to include and what to exclude. If it had been limited to real neoplasms only, a most important group of pseudotumours, which can lead to diagnostic difficulties, would have had to be omitted. In a classification of skin tumours intended to be of assistance to pathologists and their trainees, this would seem undesirable. An attempt has therefore been made to list and where possible to illustrate the more common conditions and some relatively rare ones as well. It was, however, impossible to mention, describe, and depict all these tumour-like conditions. This is particularly true of the pseudotumours, the wide range of precancerous conditions, and the hamartomas. Some selection had to be applied.

In the classification, the preferred term is given first followed, in square brackets, by synonyms in common use that were considered acceptable; certain other acceptable synonyms are referred to in the explanatory notes.

Another difficulty encountered was deciding on what clinical information, if any, should be included. Particularly in the case of skin tumours the clinical information is commonly of great value in complementing the histological information. It was felt, therefore, that some relevant clinical information should be provided, when appropriate.

Precancerous lesions and conditions

A number of precancerous lesions and conditions have been included. In a strict sense, a distinction should be made between precancerous " conditions ", e.g., xeroderma pigmentosum and precancerous " lesions ", e.g., actinic keratosis. For simplicity and ease of classification " lesions " and " conditions " have both been dealt with under one heading. Among those listed are several that will be considered by some pathologists as being not so much precancerous as already carcinoma-in-situ. Because the biological behaviour of these lesions may be quite different from that of carcinoma-in-situ in other organs, and because it also varies from one kind of lesion to another, these lesions have for the time being been included under precancerous rather than cancerous lesions.

Diagnostic procedures

Every pathologist wants to receive as large a specimen as possible—preferably the complete lesion. In widespread cutaneous involvement or where, for aesthetic reasons, large excisional biopsies are impracticable, a punch or small incisional biopsy usually suffices for diagnostic purposes. In some lesions, however, this can lead to a dangerously erroneous diagnosis. For instance, a small biopsy of a keratoacanthoma can easily lead to the wrong diagnosis of squamous cell carcinoma. Frozen section diagnosis is to be avoided, as a rule, but may be indicated in selected cases where it is necessary to differentiate a malignant melanoma from other pigmented or pseudopigmented lesions. In such cases, however, the importance of receiving a complete excisional biopsy specimen should be stressed.

For diagnostic purposes, carefully prepared thin paraffin sections from properly fixed tissue and stained with haematoxylin and eosin will usually suffice, but special staining techniques may have to be applied in particular instances. For example, there may be difficulty in distinguishing a dermatofibroma with much iron pigment from a blue naevus; an iron stain can solve this problem. To indicate the presence of mucin, it is advisable to apply several appropriate stains because some of them, particularly mucicarmine, can be very unreliable. For any of the special stains controls should always be provided.

* *
*

It should be stressed that, in general, a histological picture does not always allow the biological behaviour of a tumour to be predicted. For instance, squamous cell carcinoma arising in actinically damaged skin will rarely, if ever, lead to extensive destruction and secondary formations. A tumour of similar basic histological features but arising in scar-damaged skin may behave much more aggressively. Carcinoma of the sebaceous glands is histologically practically indistinguishable from one arising in the Meibomian glands of the eyelid, but the latter generally shows more aggressive behaviour. Malignant melanoma arising in a melanotic freckle on the face usually has a much more favourable prognosis than one arising at a different site. There are many more such examples, but it is hoped that those given will be of some guidance to the histopathologist.

HISTOLOGICAL CLASSIFICATION
OF SKIN TUMOURS

I. EPITHELIAL TUMOURS AND TUMOUR-LIKE LESIONS

A. BASAL CELL CARCINOMA

    1. Variants of basal cell carcinoma

        (a) superficial multicentric type

        (b) morphoea type

        (c) fibroepithelial

B. SQUAMOUS CELL CARCINOMA

    1. Variants of squamous cell carcinoma

        (a) adenoid squamous cell carcinoma

        (b) spindle cell type

C. METATYPICAL CARCINOMA

D. SWEAT GLAND TUMOURS AND RELATED LESIONS

    1. Benign

        (a) papillary syringadenoma [syringocystadenoma papilliferum]

        (b) papillary hidradenoma [hidradenoma papilliferum]

        (c) eccrine spiradenoma

        (d) eccrine acrospiroma [clear cell hidradenoma]

        (e) chondroid syringoma [mixed tumour, salivary gland type]

        (f) syringoma

        (g) eccrine dermal cylindroma

        (h) hidrocystoma

        (i) others

2. Malignant (sweat gland carcinoma)
   - (*a*) malignant counterparts of types I.D.1 (*a*)–(*h*)
   - (*b*) mucinous adenocarcinoma
   - (*c*) unclassified malignant sweat gland tumours

E. SEBACEOUS GLAND TUMOURS

1. Benign
   - (*a*) sebaceous adenoma

2. Malignant
   - (*a*) carcinoma of sebaceous glands
   - (*b*) carcinoma of ceruminous glands

3. Tumour-like lesions
   - (*a*) naevus sebaceus of Jadassohn
   - (*b*) adenoma sebaceum (Pringle)
   - (*c*) steatocystoma multiplex
   - (*d*) hyperplasia of sebaceous glands
   - (*e*) rhinophyma

F. TUMOURS OF HAIR FOLLICLE

1. Trichoepithelioma
2. Trichofolliculoma
3. Trichilemmoma
4. Pilomatrixoma [calcifying epithelioma of Malherbe]
5. Inverted follicular keratosis

G. PAGET'S DISEASE

1. Mammary
2. Extramammary

H. UNDIFFERENTIATED CARCINOMA

I. CYSTS

1. Keratinous cysts

(a) pilar cyst [trichilemmal, follicular, sebaceous]

(b) epidermal cyst

2. Dermoid cyst

3. Others

J. TUMOUR-LIKE LESIONS

1. Seborrhoeic keratosis

2. Keratoacanthoma

3. Benign squamous keratosis [keratotic papilloma]

4. Virus lesions

(a) verruca vulgaris

(b) verruca plana

(c) condyloma acuminatum

(d) molluscum contagiosum

5. Hamartomas

(a) naevus verrucosus

(b) naevus comedonicus

(c) others

6. Others

(a) acanthosis nigricans

(b) pseudo-epitheliomatous hyperplasia

(c) isolated dyskeratosis follicularis [warty dyskeratoma]

(d) clear cell acanthoma

K. UNCLASSIFIED

II. PRECANCEROUS LESIONS AND CONDITIONS

A. ACTINIC KERATOSIS [SOLAR, SENILE KERATOSIS]

B. RADIATION DERMATOSIS

C. BOWEN'S DISEASE

D. ERYTHROPLASIA OF QUEYRAT

E. INTRAEPIDERMAL EPITHELIOMA OF JADASSOHN

F. XERODERMA PIGMENTOSUM

G. OTHERS

III. TUMOURS AND LESIONS OF THE MELANOGENIC SYSTEM

A. BENIGN (NAEVUS)

1. Junctional naevus

2. Compound naevus

3. Intradermal naevus

4. Epithelioid and/or spindle cell naevus [juvenile melanoma]

5. Balloon cell naevus

6. Halo naevus

7. Giant pigmented naevus

8. Fibrous papule of the nose [involuting naevus]

9. Blue naevus

10. Cellular blue naevus

B. PRECANCEROUS

1. Precancerous melanosis including Hutchinson's melanotic freckle

C. MALIGNANT

1. Malignant melanoma

2. Malignant melanoma arising in precancerous melanosis, including Hutchinson's melanotic freckle

3. Malignant melanoma arising in a blue naevus

4. Malignant melanoma arising in a giant pigmented naevus

D. NON-TUMOROUS PIGMENTED LESIONS

1. Mongolian spot

2. Lentigo

3. Ephelis

IV. SOFT TISSUE TUMOURS AND TUMOUR-LIKE LESIONS

A. TUMOURS OF FIBROUS TISSUE

1. Benign
    (a) fibroma
    (b) dermatofibroma [histiocytoma, sclerosing haemangioma]

2. Malignant
    (a) dermatofibrosarcoma protuberans
    (b) fibrosarcoma

3. Tumour-like lesions
    (a) cutaneous fibrous polyp [skin tag]
    (b) hyperplastic scar
    (c) keloid
    (d) nodular fasciitis

B. TUMOURS OF FAT TISSUE

1. Benign
    (a) lipoma
    (b) angiolipoma
    (c) hibernoma

2. Malignant
    (a) liposarcoma

C. TUMOURS OF MUSCLE

1. Benign
    (a) leiomyoma

2. Malignant

   (*a*) leiomyosarcoma

D. TUMOURS OF BLOOD VESSELS

1. Benign

   (*a*) haemangioma of granulation tissue type
      [granuloma pyogenicum]

   (*b*) capillary haemangioma [juvenile haemangioma]

   (*c*) cavernous haemangioma

   (*d*) verrucous keratotic haemangioma

   (*e*) glomus tumour group

      (i) glomus tumour

      (ii) glomangioma

      (iii) angiomyoma

   (*f*) angiokeratoma

      (i) Mibelli and Fordyce types

      (ii) Fabry type [angiokeratoma corporis diffusum]

   (*g*) others

2. Malignant

   (*a*) angiosarcoma [malignant haemangioendothelioma]

   (*b*) Kaposi's sarcoma [multiple idiopathic haemorrhagic sarcoma]

3. Tumour-like lesions

   (*a*) reactive blood vessel hyperplasia

E. TUMOURS OF LYMPH VESSELS

1. Benign

   (*a*) lymphangioma

      (i) capillary lymphangioma

      (ii) cavernous lymphangioma

      (iii) cystic lymphangioma [hygroma]

2. Malignant

   (*a*) lymphangiosarcoma [malignant lymphangioendothelioma]

F. TUMOURS OF PERIPHERAL NERVES

  1. Benign
      (a) neurofibroma and plexiform neuroma
      (b) neurilemmoma [schwannoma]

  2. Malignant
      (a) malignant schwannoma
      (b) others

  3. Tumour-like lesions
      (a) traumatic neuroma
      (b) nasal glioma
      (c) cutaneous meningioma
      (d) others

G. TUMOUR-LIKE XANTHOMATOUS LESIONS

  1. Xanthoma
  2. Fibroxanthoma
  3. Atypical fibroxanthoma
  4. Juvenile xanthogranuloma [naevo-xanthoendothelioma]
  5. Reticulohistiocytic granuloma [reticulohistiocytoma]

H. MISCELLANEOUS TUMOURS AND TUMOUR-LIKE LESIONS

  1. Granular cell tumour
  2. Osteoma cutis
  3. Chondroma cutis
  4. Myxoma
  5. Cutaneous focal mucinosis
  6. Cutaneous myxoid cyst
  7. Fibrous hamartoma of infancy
  8. Recurring digital fibroma
  9. Pseudosarcoma
  10. Rheumatoid nodule

11. Pseudorheumatoid nodule [deep granuloma annulare]

12. Tumoral calcinosis

13. Others

V. TUMOURS AND TUMOUR-LIKE CONDITIONS OF THE HAEMATOPOIETIC AND LYMPHOID TISSUES

A. MYCOSIS FUNGOIDES

B. URTICARIA PIGMENTOSA [MASTOCYTOMA]

C. LEUKAEMIAS AND LYMPHOMAS

D. REACTIVE LYMPHOID HYPERPLASIA

E. BENIGN LYMPHOCYTOMA CUTIS

F. BENIGN LYMPHOCYTIC INFILTRATE OF JESSNER

G. HISTIOCYTOSIS X

H. EOSINOPHILIC GRANULOMA

VI. METASTATIC TUMOURS

VII. UNCLASSIFIED TUMOURS

CLASSIFICATION HISTOLOGIQUE
DES TUMEURS CUTANÉES

I. TUMEURS ÉPITHÉLIALES ET LÉSIONS HYPERPLASIQUES PSEUDO-TUMORALES

A. CARCINOME BASO-CELLULAIRE

1. Variétés particulières du carcinome baso-cellulaire
   - (a) superficiel et multicentrique
   - (b) sclérodermiforme [morphéiforme]
   - (c) fibro-épithélial

B. CARCINOME SPINO-CELLULAIRE

1. Variétés particulières du carcinome spino-cellulaire
   - (a) adénoïde [pseudo-glandulaire]
   - (b) carcinome à cellules fusiformes

C. CARCINOME MÉTATYPIQUE

D. TUMEURS SUDORALES ET LÉSIONS APPARENTÉES

1. Tumeurs sudorales bénignes
   - (a) syringadénome papillaire (hidradénome verruqueux fistulovégétant, syringocystadénome papillifère]
   - (b) hidradénome papillaire [hidradénome papillifère]
   - (c) spiradénome eccrine
   - (d) acrospirome eccrine [hidradénome à cellules claires, épithélioma à cellules claires]
   - (e) syringome chondroïde [tumeur dite mixte ou à stroma remanié]
   - (f) syringome
   - (g) cylindrome dermique eccrine
   - (h) hidrocystome
   - (i) autres variétés

2. Tumeurs malignes des glandes sudorales (carcinomes sudoraux ou hidradénocarcinomes)

   (a) équivalents malins des types I.D.1 (a)–(h)

   (b) adénocarcinomes mucineux

   (c) tumeurs sudorales malignes non classées

E. TUMEURS SÉBACÉES

1. Bénigne

   (a) adénome sébacé

   2. Malignes

   (a) carcinome sébacé

   (b) carcinome des glandes à cérumen

3. Lésions hyperplasiques pseudo-tumorales

   (a) naevus sébacé de Jadassohn

   (b) adénomes sébacés symétriques (Pringle)

   (c) sébocystomatose

   (d) hyperplasie sébacée

   (e) rhinophyma

F. TUMEURS PILAIRES

1. Trichoépithéliome

2. Trichofolliculome

3. Trichilemmome

4. Pilomatrixome [tumeur de Malherbe]

5. Keratosis follicularis inversa

G. MALADIE DE PAGET

1. Mammaire

2. Extramammaire

H. CARCINOME INDIFFÉRENCIÉ

I.   KYSTES

    1.   Kystes kératinisants

       (*a*)   kyste pilaire [trichilemmal, folliculaire, sébacé]

       (*b*)   kyste épidermique

    2.   Kyste dermoïde

    3.   Autres variétés

J.   LÉSIONS PSEUDO-TUMORALES

    1.   Verrue séborrhéique

    2.   Kérato-acanthome

    3.   Papillome kératosique

    4.   Lésions virales

       (*a*)   verrue vulgaire

       (*b*)   verrue plane

       (*c*)   condylome acuminé [végétation vénérienne]

       (*d*)   molluscum contagiosum

    5.   Hamartomes

       (*a*)   naevus verruqueux

       (*b*)   naevus comedonicus [naevus comedonium]

       (*c*)   autres variétés

    6.   Autres

       (*a*)   acanthosis nigricans

       (*b*)   hyperplasie pseudo-épithéliomateuse

       (*c*)   dyskeratose folliculaire isolée [dyskératome verruqueux]

       (*d*)   acanthome à cellules claires

K.   NON CLASSÉES

II.   ÉTATS PRÉCANCÉREUX

A.   KÉRATOSE ACTINIQUE [SÉNILE OU PRÉ-ÉPITHÉLIOMATEUSE]

B.   RADIODERMITES

C. MALADIE DE BOWEN

D. ERYTHROPLASIE DE QUEYRAT [MALADIE DE BOWEN DES MUQUEUSES]

E. EPITHÉLIOMA INTRAÉPIDERMIQUE DE BORST-JADASSOHN

F. XERODERMA PIGMENTOSUM

G. AUTRES

III. TUMEURS ET LÉSIONS DU SYSTÈME MÉLANOGÈNE

A. BÉNIGNES (NAEVUS)

1. Naevus jonctionnel

2. Naevus mixte

3. Naevus intradermique

4. Naevus à cellules épithéloïdes et (ou) fusiformes [mélanome juvénile de Spitz]

5. Naevus à cellules ballonnisantes

6. Naevus de Sutton

7. Naevus pigmentaire géant

8. Papule fibreuse du nez [naevus involutif]

9. Naevus bleu

10. Naevus bleu cellulaire

B. ETAT PRÉCANCÉREUX

1. Mélanose circonscrite précancéreuse de Dubreuilh

C. MALIGNES

1. Mélanome malin

2. Mélanome malin sur mélanose de Dubreuilh

3. Mélanome malin sur naevus bleu

4. Mélanome malin développé sur naevus pigmentaire géant

D. LÉSIONS PIGMENTÉES NON TUMORALES

1. Tache mongolique

2. Lentigo

3. Ephélides

IV. TUMEURS MÉSENCHYMATEUSES ET LÉSIONS PSEUDO-TUMORALES

A. TUMEURS DU TISSU CONJONCTIF

1. Bénignes

   (a) fibrome
   (b) dermatofibrome [histiocytome, histiocytofibrome]

2. Malignes

   (a) dermato-fibrosarcome de Darier et Ferrand
   (b) fibrosarcome

3. Lésions pseudo-tumorales

   (a) molluscum pendulum
   (b) cicatrice hypertrophique
   (c) chéloïde
   (d) fasciite nodulaire

B. TUMEURS DU TISSU ADIPEUX

1. Bénignes

   (a) lipome
   (b) angiolipome
   (c) hibernome

2. Maligne

   (a) lipocarsome

C. TUMEURS MUSCULAIRES

1. Bénigne

   (a) léiomyome cutané [dermatomyome]

2. Maligne

   (a) léiomyosarcome

D. TUMEURS DES VAISSEAUX SANGUINS

1. Bénignes

   (a) hémangiome acquis inflammatoire [granulome pyogénique ou télangiectasique, "botryomycome"]

   (b) hémangiome capillaire [hémangiome juvénile]

   (c) hémangiome caverneux

   (d) hémangiome kératosique verruqueux [angiome kératosique]

   (e) groupe des tumeurs glomiques

      (i) tumeur glomique

      (ii) glomangiome

      (iii) angiomyome

   (f) angiokératome

      (i) de Mibelli et de Fordyce

      (ii) de Fabry

   (g) autres variétés

2. Malignes

   (a) angiosarcome [hémangioendothéliome malin

   (b) maladie de Kaposi

3. Etat pseudo-tumoral

   (a) hyperplasie vasculo-sanguine réactionnelle

E. TUMEURS DES VAISSEAUX LYMPHATIQUES

1. Bénignes

   (a) lymphangiome

      (i) capillaire

      (ii) caverneux

      (iii) kystique

2. Maligne

   (a) lymphangiosarcome [lymphangioendothéliome malin]

F.   TUMEURS DES NERFS PÉRIPHÉRIQUES

1. Bénignes

   (*a*)   neurofibrome et névrome plexiforme

   (*b*)   neurilemmome [schwannome]

2. Malignes

   (*a*)   schwannome malin

   (*b*)   autres variétés

3. Etats pseudo-tumoraux

   (*a*)   névrome post-traumatique

   (*b*)   gliome nasal

   (*c*)   méningiome cutané

   (*d*)   autres variétés

G.   LÉSIONS XANTHOMATEUSES PSEUDO-TUMORALES

1. Xanthome

2. Fibroxanthome

3. Fibroxanthome atypique

4. Xanthogranulome juvénile [naevo-xantho-endothéliome]

5. Granulome réticulo-histiocytaire [reticulohistiocytome]

H.   TUMEURS ET LÉSIONS PSEUDO-TUMORALES VARIÉES

1. Tumeurs à cellules granuleuses d'Abrikossoff

2. Ostéome cutané

3. Chondrome cutané

4. Myxome

5. Mucinose focale cutanée

6. Kyste mucoïde cutané [kyste dit synovial]

7. Hamartome fibreux infantile

8. Fibrome digital récidivant

9. Pseudosarcome

10. Nodule rhumatismal juxta-articulaire

11. Granulome annulaire profond
12. Calcinose pseudo-tumorale
13. Autres variétés

V. TUMEURS ET ÉTATS PSEUDO-TUMORAUX DES TISSUS HÉMATOPOIÉTIQUE ET LYMPHOÏDE

A. MYCOSIS FONGOÏDE

B. URTICAIRE PIGMENTAIRE [MASTOCYTOME]

C. LEUCÉMIES CUTANÉES ET RÉTICULOSES MALIGNES

D. HYPERPLASIE LYMPHOÏDE RÉACTIONNELLE

E. LYMPHOCYTOME CUTANÉ BÉNIN

F. INFILTRATION LYMPHOCYTAIRE BÉNIGNE DE JESSNER

G. HISTIOCYTOSIS-X

H. GRANULOME ÉOSINOPHILE

VI. TUMEURS MÉTASTATIQUES

VII. TUMEURS NON CLASSÉES

ГИСТОЛОГИЧЕСКАЯ КЛАССИФИКАЦИЯ
ОПУХОЛЕЙ КОЖИ

I. ЭПИТЕЛИАЛЬНЫЕ ОПУХОЛИ
И ОПУХОЛЕПОДОБНЫЕ ПОРАЖЕНИЯ

A. Базальноклеточный рак

1. Варианты базальноклеточного рака
   (*a*) Поверхностный мультицентрический
   (*b*) Тип морфеа
   (*c*) Фибро–эпителиальный

B. Плоскоклеточный рак

1. Варианты плоскоклеточного рака
   (*a*) Аденоидный плоскоклеточный рак
   (*b*) Веретеноклеточный тип

C. Метатипичный рак

D. Опухоли потовых желез и родственные поражения

1. Доброкачественные
   (*a*) Папиллярная сирингаденома
   (*b*) Папиллярная гидроаденома
   (*c*) Эккринная спираденома
   (*d*) Эккринная акроспирома
   (*e*) Хондроидная сирингома [смешанная опухоль из слюнных желез]
   (*f*) Сирингома
   (*g*) Эккринная кожная цилиндрома
   (*h*) Гидроцистома [потовая киста]
   (*i*) Другие

2. Злокачественные (рак потовых желез)

   (*a*) Злокачественные аналоги опухолей, указанных в I.D.1 (*a*)–(*h*)

   (*b*) Слизистая аденокарцинома

   (*c*) Неклассифицируемые злокачественные опухоли потовых желез

E. Опухоли сальных желез

   1. Доброкачественные

      (*a*) Аденома сальных желез

   2. Злокачественные

      (*a*) Рак сальных желез

      (*b*) Рак серных желез

   3. Опухолеподобные поражения

      (*a*) Невус сальных желез (Ядассона)

      (*b*) «Аденома» сальных желез (Прингле)

      (*c*) Сложная жировая киста

      (*d*) Гиперплазия сальных желез

      (*e*) Ринофима

F. Опухоли из волосяного фолликула

   1. Трихоэпителиома

   2. Трихофолликулома

   3. Трихолеммома

   4. Опухоль волосяного матрикса [обызвествленная эпителиома Малерба]

   5. Инвертирующий фолликулярный кератоз

G. Болезнь Педжета

   1. Молочной железы

   2. Прочих локализаций

H. Недифференцированный рак

I. Кисты

    1. Кератиновые кисты

        (*a*) Волосяный кист [фолликулярный, сальный]

        (*b*) Эпидермальный кист

    2. Дермоидный кист

    3. Другие

J. Опухолеподобные поражения

    1. Себоррейный кератоз

    2. Кератоакантома

    3. Доброкачественный плоскоклеточный кератоз [папиллома с кератозом]

    4. Вирусные поражения

        (*a*) Вульгарная бородавка

        (*b*) Плоская бородавка

        (*c*) Острокопытная кондилома

        (*d*) Контагиозный моллюск

    5. Гамартомы

        (*a*) Бородавчатый невус

        (*b*) Угревидный невус

        (*c*) Другие

    6. Другие

        (*a*) Акантозис нигриканс

        (*b*) Псевдо–эпителиоматозная гиперплазия

        (*c*) Изолированный фолликулярный дискератоз

        (*d*) Светлоклеточная акантома

K. Неклассифицированные

II. ПРЕДРАКОВЫЕ СОСТОЯНИЯ

A. Актинический кератоз [сенильный кератоз]

B. Радиационный дерматоз

C. Болезнь Боуэна

D. Эритроплазия Кейра

E. Внутридермальная эпителиома Ядассона

F. Пигментная ксеродерма

G. Другие

III. ОПУХОЛИ И ПОРАЖЕНИЯ МЕЛАНОГЕНЕТИЧЕСКОЙ СИСТЕМЫ

A. Доброкачественные (невусы)

1. Пограничный невус
2. Сложный невус
3. Внутридермальный невус
4. Эпителиоид и/или вертеноклеточный невус
5. Невус из баллонообразных клеток
6. Галоневус
7. Гигантский пигментированный невус
8. Фиброзная папула носа [инволюционный невус]
9. Голубой невус
10. Клеточный голубой невус

B. Предраковые изменения

1. Предраковый меланоз, меланотическое пятно Хатчинсона

C. Злокачественные

1. Злокачественная меланома
2. Злокачественная меланома, возникшая из предракового меланоза, включая меланотическое пятно Хатчинсона
3. Злокачественная меланома, возникшая из голубого невуса
4. Злокачественная меланома, возникшая из гигантского пигментированного невуса

D. Неопухолевые пигментные поражения

   1. Монгольское пятно

   2. Лентиго

   3. Эфелид

IV. ОПУХОЛИ МЯГКИХ ТКАНЕЙ И ОПУХОЛЕПОДОБНЫЕ ПОРАЖЕНИЯ

A. Опухоли фиброзной ткани

   1. Доброкачественные

      (*a*) Фиброма

      (*b*) Дерматофиброма [гистиоцитома, склерозирующая гемангиома]

   2. Злокачественные

      (*a*) Дерматофибросаркома протуберанс

      (*b*) Фибросаркома

   3. Опухолеподобные поражения

      (*a*) Фиброзный полип кожи

      (*b*) Гиперпластический рубец

      (*c*) Келоид

      (*d*) Узловатый фасцит

B. Опухоли жировой ткани

   1. Доброкачественные

      (*a*) Липома

      (*b*) Ангиолипома

      (*c*) Гибернома

   2. Злокачественные

      (*a*) Липосаркома

C. Опухоли мышц

   1. Доброкачественные

      (*a*) Лейомиома

2. Злокачественные

(*a*) Лейомиосаркома

D. Опухоли кровеносных сосудов

1. Доброкачественные

(*a*) Гемангиома грануляционнотканного типа [пиогенная гранулома]

(*b*) Капиллярная гемангиома [ювенильная гемангиома]

(*c*) Кавернозная гемангиома

(*d*) Бородавчатая кератотическая гемангиома

(*e*) Группа гломических опухолей

    i. гломическая опухоль

    ii. гломангиома

    iii. ангиомиома

(*f*) Ангиокератома

    i. типы Мибелли и Фордайса

    ii. тип Фабри

(*g*) Другие

2. Злокачественные

(*a*) Ангиосаркома [злокачественная гемангиоэндотелиома]

(*b*) Саркома Капоши

3. Опухолеподобные поражения

(*a*) Реактивная сосудистая гиперплазия

E. Опухоли лимфатических сосудов

1. Доброкачественные

(*a*) Лимфангиома

    i. капиллярная лимфангиома

    ii. кавернозная лимфангиома

    iii. кистовидная лимфангиома [гигрома]

2. Злокачественные

(*a*) Лимфангиосаркома [злокачественная лимфангио-эндотелиома]

F. Опухоли периферических нервов

1. Доброкачественные

   (*a*) Нейрофиброма и неврома в виде сплетения

   (*b*) Нейролеммома [шваннома]

2. Злокачественные

   (*a*) Злокачественная шваннома

   (*b*) Другие

3. Опухолеподобные поражения

   (*a*) Травматическая неврома

   (*b*) Глиома носа

   (*c*) Менингиома кожи

   (*d*) Другие

G. Опухолеподобные ксантоматозные поражения

1. Ксантома

2. Фиброксантома

3. Атипичная фиброксантома

4. Ювенильная ксантогранулема [ксантоэндотелиома]

5. Ретикулогистиоцитарная гранулема [ретикулогистиоцитома]

H. Прочие опухоли и опухолеподобные поражения

1. Зернисто–клеточная опухоль

2. Остеома кожи

3. Хондрома кожи

4. Миксома

5. Очаговое ослизнение кожи

6. Миксоидная киста кожи

7. Фиброзная гамартома младенцев

8. Рецидивирующая фиброма пальцев

9. Псевдосаркома

10. Ревматоидный узелок

11. Псевдоревматоидный узелок (глубокая кольцевидная гранулема)

12. Опухолевый кальциноз

13. Другие

V. ОПУХОЛИ И ОПУХОЛЕПОДОБНЫЕ ИЗМЕНЕНИЯ ГЕМАТОПОЭТИЧЕСКОЙ И ЛИМФОИДНОЙ ТКАНЕЙ

A. Грибовидный микоз

B. Пигментная крапивница (мастоцитома)

C. Лейкозы

D. Реактивная лимфоидная гиперплазия

E. Доброкачественная лимфоцитома кожи

F. Доброкачественный лимфоцитарный инфильтрат Джесснера

G. Гистиоцитоз «Х»

H. Эозинофильная гранулема

VI. МЕТАСТАТИЧЕСКИЕ ОПУХОЛИ

VII. НЕКЛАССИФИЦИРУЕМЫЕ ОПУХОЛИ

CLASIFICACION HISTOLOGICA
DE LOS TUMORES CUTANEOS

I. TUMORES EPITELIALES Y LESIONES SEUDOTUMORALES

A. CARCINOMA BASOCELULAR

    1. Variantes de carcinoma basocelular

       (*a*) multicéntrico superficial

       (*b*) tipo morfea

       (*c*) fibroepitelial

B. CARCINOMA ESPINOCELULAR

    1. Variantes de carcinoma espinocelular

       (*a*) carcinoma espinocelular adenoide

       (*b*) tipo de células fusiformes

C. CARCINOMA METATÍPICO

D. TUMORES DE LAS GLÁNDULAS SUDORÍPARAS Y LESIONES AFINES

    1. Benignos

       (*a*) siringoadenoma papilar [siringocistoadenoma papilliferum]

       (*b*) hidradenoma papilar

       (*c*) espiradenoma ecrino

       (*d*) acrospiroma ecrino [hidradenoma de células claras]

       (*e*) siringoma condroide [tumor mixto, tipo glándula salival]

       (*f*) siringoma

       (*g*) cilindroma dérmico ecrino

       (*h*) hidrocistoma

       (*i*) otros

2. Maligno (carcinoma de las glándulas sudoríparas)

(a) equivalentes malignos de los tipos I.D.1 (a)–(h)

(b) adenocarcinoma mucinoso

(c) tumores malignos no clasificados de las glándulas sudoríparas

E. TUMORES DE LAS GLÁNDULAS SEBÁCEAS

1. Benignos

(a) adenoma sebáceo

2. Malignos

(a) carcinoma de las glándulas sebáceas

(b) carcinoma de las glándulas ceruminosas

3. Lesiones seudotumorales

(a) nevo sebáceo de Jadassohn

(b) adenoma sebáceo (Pringle)

(c) esteatocistoma múltiple

(d) hiperplasia de las glándulas sebáce

(e) rinofima

F. TUMORES DEL FOLÍCULO PILOSO

1. Tricoepitelioma

2. Tricofoliculoma

3. Tricolemoma

4. Pilomatrixoma [epitelioma calcificante de Malherbe]

5. Queratosis folicular invertida

G. ENFERMEDAD DE PAGET

1. Mamaria

2. Extramamaria

H. CARCINOMA INDIFERENCIADO

I.   QUISTES

    1.   Quistes queratinosos

        (*a*)   quiste piloso [tricolemal, folicular, sebáceo]

        (*b*)   quiste epidérmico

    2.   Quiste dermoide

    3.   Otros

J.   LESIONES SEUDOTUMORALES

    1.   Queratosis seborréica

    2.   Queratoacantoma

    3.   Queratosis escamosa benigna [papiloma queratósico]

    4.   Lesiones virales

        (*a*)   verruga vulgar

        (*b*)   verruga plana

        (*c*)   condiloma acuminado

        (*d*)   molusco contagioso

    5.   Hamartomas

        (*a*)   nevo verrugoso

        (*b*)   nevo comedónico

        (*c*)   otros

    6.   Otros

        (*a*)   acantosis nigricans

        (*b*)   hiperplasia seudoepiteliomatosa

        (*c*)   disqueratosis folicular aislada [disqueratoma verrugoso]

        (*d*)   acantoma de células claras

K.   SIN CLASIFICAR

II.   ENFERMEDADES PRECANCEROSAS

A.   QUERATOSIS ACTÍNICA [QUERATOSIS SOLAR, QUERATOSIS SENIL]

B.   DERMATOSIS POR IRRADIACIÓN

C. ENFERMEDAD DE BOWEN

D. ERITROPLASIA DE QUEYRAT

E. EPITELIOMA INTRAEPIDÉRMICO DE JADASSOHN

F. XERODERMA PIGMENTOSO

G. OTROS

III. TUMORES Y LESIONES DEL SISTEMA MELANOGENO

A. BENIGNOS (NEVOS)

1. Nevo de unión
2. Nevo compuesto
3. Nevo intradérmico
4. Nevo epitelioide y/o fusocelular [melanoma juvenil]
5. Nevo de células globulosas
6. Nevo de halo
7. Nevo pigmentado gigante
8. Pápula fibrosa de la nariz [nevo en involución]
9. Nevo azul
10. Nevo azul celular

B. PRECANCEROSOS

1. Melanosis precancerosa, con inclusión de la peca melanótica de Hutchinson

C. MALIGNOS

1. Melanoma maligno
2. Melanoma maligno en una melanosis precancerosa con inclusión de la peca melanótica de Hutchinson
3. Melanoma maligno originado en un nevo azul
4. Melanoma maligno originado en un nevo pigmentado gigante

D. LESIONES PIGMENTADAS NO TUMORALES

1. Mancha mongólica
2. Léntigo
3. Efélide

IV. TUMORES Y LESIONES SEUDOTUMORALES DE LOS TEJIDOS BLANDOS

A. TUMORES DEL TEJIDO FIBROSO

1. Benignos
    (*a*) fibroma
    (*b*) dermatofibroma [histiocitoma, hemangioma esclerosante]

2. Malignos
    (*a*) dermatofibrosarcoma protuberante
    (*b*) fibrosarcoma

3. Lesiones seudotumorales
    (*a*) pólipo fibroso cutáneo
    (*b*) cicatriz hiperplásica
    (*c*) queloide
    (*d*) fascitis nodular

B. TUMORES DEL TEJIDO ADIPOSO

1. Benignos
    (*a*) lipoma
    (*b*) angiolipoma
    (*c*) hibernoma

2. Malignos
    (*a*) liposarcoma

C. TUMORES DEL MÚSCULO

1. Benignos
    (*a*) leiomioma

2. Malignos

    (a) leiomiosarcoma

D. TUMORES DE LOS VASOS SANGUÍNEOS

  1. Benignos

    (a) hemangioma, tipo tejido de granulación [granuloma piogénico]

    (b) hemangioma capilar [hemangioma juvenil]

    (c) hemangioma cavernoso

    (d) hemangioma verrugoso queratósico

    (e) grupo de tumores glómicos

      (i) tumor glómico

      (ii) glomangioma

      (iii) angiomioma

    (f) angioqueratoma

      (i) tipos Mibelli y Fordyce

      (ii) tipo Fabry [angioqueratoma corporis diffusum]

    (g) otros

  2. Malignos

    (a) angiosarcoma [hemangioendotelioma maligno]

    (b) sarcoma de Kaposi [sarcoma hemorrágico idiopático multiple]

  3. Lesiones seudotumorales

    Hiperplasia vascular reactiva

E. TUMORES DE LOS VASOS LINFÁTICOS

  1. Benignos

    (a) linfangioma

      (i) capilar

      (ii) cavernoso

      (iii) quistico (higroma)

  2. Malignos

    (a) linfangiosarcoma [linfangioendotelioma maligno]

F. TUMORES DE LOS NERVIOS PERIFÉRICOS

1. Benignos

(a) neurofibroma y neuroma plexiforme

(b) neurilemoma [schwannoma]

2. Malignos

(a) schwannoma maligno

(b) otros

3. Lesiones seudotumorales

(a) neuroma traumático

(b) glioma nasal

(c) meningioma cutáneo

(d) otros

G. LESIONES XANTOMATOSAS SEUDOTUMORALES

1. Xantoma

2. Fibroxantoma

3. Fibroxantoma atípico

4. Xantogranuloma juvenil [nevoxantoendotelioma]

5. Granuloma reticulohistiocitario [reticulohistiocitoma]

H. OTROS TUMORES Y LESIONES SEUDOTUMORALES

1. Tumor de células granulosas

2. Osteoma cutáneo

3. Condroma cutáneo

4. Mixoma

5. Mucinosis focal cutánea

6. Quiste mixoide cutáneo

7. Hamartoma fibrosa

8. Fibroma recurrente del dedo

9. Seudosarcoma

10. Nódulo reumatoide

11. Nódulo seudorreumático [granuloma anular profundo]
12. Calcinosis tumoral
13. Otros

V. TUMORES Y LESIONES SEUDOTUMORALES DE LOS TEJIDOS HEMATOPOYETICO Y LINFOIDE

A. MICOSIS FUNGOIDE

B. URTICARIA PIGMENTOSA [MASTOCITOMA]

C. LEUCEMIAS Y LINFOMAS

D. HIPERPLASIA LINFOIDE REACTIVA

E. LINFOCITOMA CUTÁNEO BENIGNO

F. INFILTRADO LINFOCÍTICO BENIGNO DE JESSNER

G. HISTIOCITOSIS X

H. GRANULOMA EOSINÓFILO

VI. TUMORES METASTASICOS

VII. TUMORES NO CLASIFICADOS

DEFINITIONS
AND EXPLANATORY NOTES

I. EPITHELIAL TUMOURS AND TUMOUR-LIKE LESIONS

A. BASAL CELL CARCINOMA (Fig. 1-9)

A locally invasive, slowly spreading tumour, which rarely metastasizes, arising in the epidermis or hair follicles and in which, in particular, the peripheral cells usually simulate the basal cells of the epidermis.

These tumours can arise anywhere on the body but particularly in sites exposed to the sun, especially on the face in elderly persons. Exceptions are those arising in the " naevoid basal cell carcinoma syndrome " in which multiple basal cell carcinomas, cysts of the jaws, bifid ribs, and other changes occur. However, on the basis of the histological appearance alone the naevoid cannot be distinguished from an ordinary basal cell carcinoma.

The histological pattern shows an extraordinary variety and solid, cystic, and adenoid types can be recognized. Areas of keratinization can occur and melanin pigment may be present. Some show areas of sebaceous differentiation of varying extent. Any of the different types can occur singly or in combination with one or more of the others in one and the same lesion. Clinically they cannot be distinguished. This general statement does not hold for the following variants which exhibit clinical and/or histological differences.

1. *Variants of basal cell carcinoma*

(a) *Superficial multicentric type* (Fig. 7)

A basal cell carcinoma composed of multiple foci or buds of tumour cells, which occur at intervals along the epidermis and extend into the adjacent corium.

When left alone over a long period some of the extensions can penetrate deeper into the corium and the " superficial " aspect becomes lost. This variant of basal cell carcinoma commonly occurs on the trunk.

(b) *Morphoea type* (Fig. 8)

A basal cell carcinoma with nests of tumour cells, usually small strands, seemingly separated and surrounded by a desmoplastic, often cicatrical stroma.

When these histological characteristics occur in the deeper parts of what otherwise is a typical basal cell carcinoma, the tumours have a much greater tendency to recur and/or progress.

(c) *Fibroepithelial type* (Fig. 9)

A typically elevated tumour that contains branching and anastomosing cords of atypical basal cells surrounding islands of stroma.

Although this type of tumour was initially described as " premalignant ", it is considered preferable to classify it as a distinct form of basal cell carcinoma.

B. SQUAMOUS CELL CARCINOMA (Fig. 10-15)

An invasive tumour that shows evidence of squamous differentiation.

Histologically squamous cell carcinomas may show considerable variation. Infiltration into the corium and eventually into the subcutis takes place, with finger-like projections extending like the roots of a tree. The cells usually show great variation in size and staining properties and dyskeratotic and parakeratotic cells, sometimes arranged in a whorled fashion, are characteristic. The nuclei are prominent and vary in size and staining properties. Mitotic figures are usually easy to find and occasionally may be very numerous and pronounced. In such cases the parakeratotic changes may be less noticeable or even absent. Cellular bridges may be found quite easily or may be very difficult to demonstrate, depending on the degree of differentiation.

The tumours may arise on any part of the body, but are particularly liable to occur on parts exposed to the sun. A clinical distinction should be made between squamous cell carcinomas arising in actinic keratosis and those arising in scar tissue due to burns, mechanical injury or chronic, more or less specific inflammation (Marjolin's ulcer, lupus vulgaris, etc.), although histologically there are no obvious differences. In contrast to tumours in the latter group, however, those arising in sun-damaged skin rarely, if ever, metastasize. Only a small percentage of the adenoid squamous cell carcinomas metastasize.

1. *Variants of squamous cell carcinoma*

(a) *Adenoid squamous cell carcinoma* (Fig. 12-13)

A tumour with a glandular or acinar pattern and also containing definite squamous cells.

Acantholysis is frequently present in the glandular parts. This tumour has been called adenoacanthoma.

Some carcinomas arising from glandular structures but having numerous squamous cells can lead to confusing histological patterns. The application of mucin and/or mucin-keratin stains may help to differentiate these tumours.

(b) *Spindle cell type* (Fig. 14)

An uncommon type of squamous cell carcinoma in which the cells have a spindle shape.

There may be considerable difficulty in distinguishing these from pseudosarcoma, true sarcoma, or even spindle cell malignant melanoma.

Combined forms of the different histological types may occur.

C.   METATYPICAL CARCINOMA (Fig. 16-18)

Tumours in which either the cell type and/or the arrangement of the cells causes difficulty in deciding between basal cell carcinoma or squamous cell carcinoma; they have occasionally been classified as basosquamous cell carcinomas.

After previous radiation, basal cell carcinomas sometimes show a pattern of growth in which the cells tend to be polygonal with acidophilic cytoplasm (Fig. 16). These tumours show a high invasive potential and they occasionally metastasize. They should be classified as metatypical. They have also been called " intermediate " carcinomas.

In other metatypical carcinomas the growth pattern is like that of a basal cell carcinoma but the individual cells have a more squamous appearance and many show parakeratosis (Fig. 17-18). Although different from the previous group they are also best classified as metatypical.

D.   SWEAT GLAND TUMOURS AND RELATED LESIONS

Tumours and tumour-like lesions arising from or resembling any part of the eccrine or apocrine sweat gland structures.

There are a number of lesions derived from sweat gland structures that are not known for certain to be true neoplasms; some are more likely to be hamartomatous in nature. For convenience these have been included in this part of the classification.

1. *Benign sweat gland tumours*

(a) *Papillary syringadenoma* [*syringocystadenoma papilliferum*] (Fig. 19-20)

A tumour in which the overlying epidermis shows some papillomatosis with several cystic extensions into the corium. Numerous epithelial projections, commonly villus-like, extend into the cystic areas. The epithelial lining consists of two rows of cells, tall columnar cells lining the inside and small cuboidal cells with deeply staining nuclei on the dermal side. The stroma of the villi nearly always contain a dense infiltrate of plasma cells.

This tumour frequently arises as a single lesion on the scalp.

(b) *Papillary hidradenoma* [*hidradenoma papilliferum*] (Fig. 21-22)

A tumour located in the dermis under a normal epidermis and composed of an intricate lace-like pattern of papillae, which are covered with one or two layers of epithelium. The superficial cells resembling apocrine epithelium are either columnar with decapitation features or larger plump acidophilic cells. Plasma cells are sparse or absent.

This is usually only a small lesion and occurs solely in women in the skin of the genital area (labia majora, perianal, and perineal region).

(c) *Eccrine spiradenoma* (Fig. 23-24)

A tumour that resembles the secretory segment of the sweat gland apparatus and consists of a mixture of small cells with round uniform nuclei and slightly larger cells with paler nuclei.

An eccrine spiradenoma is commonly surrounded by a thin fibrous capsule. The arrangement may be without a pattern but sometimes glandular structures are present. Irregular cystic spaces, haemorrhage, and marked oedema occur. This is a painful circumscribed nodule occurring in the dermis, usually as a single lesion.

(d) *Eccrine acrospiroma* [*clear cell hidradenoma, clear cell epithelioma*] (Fig. 25-29)

A tumour that mimics the structure of the eccrine duct, including the acral segment surrounding the pore.

Histologically the tumour is usually circumscribed but not encapsulated and it is commonly multilobular. It may be solid or partly cystic. The solid part consists of cells with a biphasic pattern. They are usually round or polygonal, occasionally elongated, and many have either a clear or eosinophilic cytoplasm. Some of the tumours are entirely composed of clear cells, which contain a large amount of glycogen. Many tumours show attempted ductal formation. Occasionally these tumours undergo malignant change. They usually occur singly and may be located anywhere on the body. In some instances they show oozing or draining on the surface. Those tumours occurring on the sole of the foot have been called eccrine poromas.

(e)　Chondroid syringoma [mixed tumour, salivary gland type] (Fig. 30-31)

A tumour that appears to be composed of a mixture of epithelial and mesenchymal tissues.

The tumour exhibits irregular ducts and sometimes acini that mimic sweat gland structures as well as solid nests of epithelial cells, which extend into the surrounding matrix where they assume the appearance of chondrocytes. The chondroid matrix is rich in sulfated acid mucopolysaccharide and is similar to that seen in cartilage.

Chondroid syringomas can occur in all areas of the body but are most common in the region of the head. They are usually relatively small and painless and situated in the dermis, and they are circumscribed but not encapsulated.

A malignant form (chondroid syringocarcinoma), although rare, has been described.

(f)　Syringoma (Fig. 32-33)

A tumour characterized by groups of epithelial cells in duct-like formation connecting with small cavities lined by cuboidal cells. Often a configuration is found in which the epithelial cells are arranged in nests with tails separated by a fibrous stroma.

This tumour may occur as a single papule or as multiple papules involving many areas of the body. It is sometimes confined to the eyelids.

(g)　Eccrine dermal cylindroma (Fig. 34-35)

A characteristically lobulated tumour composed of epithelial cell nests surrounded by a hyaline membrane and embedded in a loose stroma.

Hyalin may be present among the epithelial cells. Within the tumour cells are secretory vacuoles containing acid mucopolysaccharide and pockets of similar substances are present in the hyaline membrane.

The term "eccrine" is controversial, some authors believing that the lesion arises from apocrine glands. This is not confirmed, however, by electron microscopy. The opinion has also been expressed that these tumours may arise from the pilar complex.

Eccrine dermal cylindroma occurs mainly on the scalp and face and in rare instances elsewhere on the body. It is commonly multiple and the variation in size is very considerable. The multiple form on the scalp has been called "turban tumour".

(h) *Hidrocystoma* (Fig. 36)

A unilocular or multilocular cystic structure lined by columnar or cuboidal epithelium resting on an outer layer of flattened cells.

The epithelium has an apocrine-like structure and occasionally exhibits papillary infoldings. Pigment granules, probably lipofuscin, are sometimes present in the cytoplasm. The lumen may contain proteinaceous secretory material. The lesions usually occur singly but a rare form with closely approximated deep-seated vesicles has been described.

(i) *Others*

Occasionally lesions are encountered that are apparently of sweat gland origin but lack the characteristic features described above. Many of these are likely to be hamartomas but it is better to classify them as variants of sweat gland adenoma.

2. *Malignant (sweat gland carcinoma)* (Fig. 37-39)

(a) *Malignant counterparts of types I.D.1 (a)–(h)*

Malignant variants can be designated as such when recognizably derived from one of the above types (e.g., malignant eccrine acrospiroma) or by the addition of the suffix carcinoma (e.g., chondroid syringo-carcinoma).

(b) *Mucinous adenocarcinoma* [*adenocystic carcinoma*] (Fig. 37-38)

A malignant epithelial tumour secreting abundant mucin.

Histologically it is characterized by nests of solid and glandular epithelium, surrounded by a sea of mucin; the nests are usually small. Some cells contain mucin. Histochemically the mucin is mostly sialomucin.

The tumour tends to ulcerate and recur but rarely to metastasize.

(c) Unclassified malignant sweat gland tumours (Fig. 39)

These are malignant sweat gland tumours that cannot be placed in the above categories.

Rarely sweat gland carcinomas may contain melanin pigment and melanocytes may even be present in metastases of such tumours.

E.   SEBACEOUS GLAND TUMOURS

1.   *Benign*

(a) Sebaceous adenoma (Fig. 40)

A tumour that is subdivided into many sebaceous gland-like lobules.

The lesions usually occur in persons past middle age, the most common site being the face.

2.   *Malignant*

(a) Carcinoma of sebaceous glands [sebaceous adenocarcinoma] (Fig. 41-42)

A malignant lipid-secreting tumour of sebaceous gland epithelium.

This tumour is composed of ill-defined lobules that vary greatly in size or of diffuse masses of cells that can be rather poorly differentiated. Variable numbers of recognizable sebaceous cells serve to identify the tumour. Pleomorphism and polychromasia of both cells and nuclei are usually striking. These are quite rare tumours which may occur anywhere on the body except the palms and soles. Many of the tumours are ulcerated.
They should be distinguished from basal cell carcinomas showing areas of sebaceous differentiation (Fig. 3-4).
Carcinomas of the Meibomian glands of the eyelids (Fig. 42) are essentially similar to other sebaceous gland carcinomas. However, these tumours behave in a much more aggressive manner.

(b) Carcinoma of ceruminous glands

A malignant tumour of ceruminous glands.

This is a rare tumour that arises in the skin of the external meatus of the ear and has histological features resembling an adenocarcinoma with varying stages of differentiation. A brown pigment, probably lipofuscin, can be identified in the cells of some of these tumours.

3.   Tumour-like lesions

(a) Naevus sebaceus of Jadassohn (Fig. 43)

A lesion characterized by hyperplasia of immature sebaceous glands and pilar structures. The overlying epidermis shows papillary acanthosis.

The lesion occurs mainly on the scalp or face and may be present at birth.

(b) Adenoma sebaceum (Pringle)

This lesion is characterized by fibrosis and dilatation of capillaries in the presence of generally atrophic sebaceous glands.

The condition occurs as part of the tuberous sclerosis complex and takes the form of symmetrically distributed small lesions on the face. The name is somewhat of a misnomer.

(c) Steatocystoma multiplex

A condition characterized by multiple small lesions, usually on the trunk, and each consisting of a cystic area lined by cuboidal and flattened epithelium, sometimes showing sebaceous cells in the wall.

(d) Hyperplasia of sebaceous glands

A lesion composed of greatly enlarged fully mature sebaceous glands arranged around a central duct into which they drain. Sometimes several ducts are present in one and the same lesion, each with its own sebaceous glands.

This lesion is commonly seen on the face, particularly on the forehead, in elderly persons and for that reason is also called " senile sebaceous hyperplasia ".

(e) Rhinophyma

A hyperplasia of sebaceous glands with increased vascularity and chronic inflammation. It is confined to the nose.

F. TUMOURS OF HAIR FOLLICLE

1. *Trichoepithelioma* (Fig. 44-45)

> A tumour containing multiple horn cysts simulating to a varying degree abortive pilar structures which may be connected by epithelial tracts.

The presence of epithelial tracts is most striking when the lesion is solitary. The tumours are usually well circumscribed and keratinization is abrupt. In addition, a foreign-body giant cell reaction and calcium deposits may be present.

Confusion between trichoepithelioma and basal cell carcinoma with more keratinization than usual can occur.

This tumour occurs in two forms; one is an inherited form in which multiple lesions (epithelioma adenoides cysticum) occur mainly on the face but sometimes also on the scalp, the neck and the upper trunk; the other is a solitary lesion, which can occur anywhere on the body, although again the face is the most common site, and it appears in later life.

2. *Trichofolliculoma* (Fig. 46)

> A lesion in which an opening in the epidermis leads to a cystic space lined by squamous epithelium with abortive hair follicles in varying stages of development. It is typically a solitary lesion occurring mainly on the face and occasionally on the scalp or in the neck.

The lesion is probably more of a hamartoma than a true neoplasm, but for convenience it is classified under the hair follicle tumours.

3. *Trichilemmoma* (Fig. 47)

> Tumours composed of solid masses of clear cuboidal to polygonal cells with sharply defined cell borders. The cytoplasm contains large amounts of glycogen. The tumour is well demarcated from the surrounding corium and is continuous with the epidermis. The cell masses are usually partly separated by thin strands of fibrous stroma resulting in a somewhat lobulated appearance. In the centre of the cell masses thin cores of keratin are usually present, reminiscent of the core of hair shafts. The surrounding epidermis commonly shows acanthosis.

These small lesions most commonly occur on the head.

4. *Pilomatrixoma* [*calcifying epithelioma of Malherbe*] (Fig. 48-50)

> A benign tumour containing cells simulating those of basal cell carcinoma as well as characteristic eosinophilic " ghost cells ".

This is a well-demarcated but not always encapsulated lesion, localized in the lower corium with extension into the subcutaneous fat. Irregular masses of epithelial cells are embedded in a fairly loose connective tissue stroma. The cells are characteristically of two types: one type is basophilic and shows a resemblance to the cells of basal cell carcinoma, the other cells are widely known as " ghost cells ". Irregular masses of calcification are commonly but not always present and lesions of longer standing can show ossification in the stroma. Areas of keratinization are common. The calcium deposits may be present as fine " dust " and/or form larger aggregates.

It is a solitary lesion which can reach considerable size and occurs mainly on the face or upper extremities. It can be present at any age.

5. *Inverted follicular keratosis* (Fig. 51-52)

A cellular epithelial mass of keratinocytes ranging in appearance from those just above the basal layer to mature squamous cells. These cells in transition often occur in small clusters or " squamous eddies " among the less mature cells. The mass of cells sometimes has a central crypt and may show more than one broad projection into the dermis. It is covered laterally by the extension upward of the normal epidermis, which gives the impression of inversion. The base of the lesion is usually fairly well defined and the surface may be covered by a thick verrucous horn of keratin and parakeratin. The lesion is benign but may recur.

This lesion is usually a solitary papule or nodule projecting from the surface of the skin. The face is a common site.

G. PAGET'S DISEASE

A lesion characterized by the presence along the basal margin or through the epidermis or mucosa of large pale-staining cells with large but sometimes compressed vesicular nuclei (" Paget " cells). The cells may occur singly or in groups and compress the epidermal cells.

1. *Mammary*

2. *Extramammary* (Fig. 53-54)

An underlying duct carcinoma is nearly always present in Paget's disease of the nipple but does not occur nearly so commonly in the sweat-gland ducts of the extramammary form. The origin of the Paget cells is still in dispute. This is not the place to enter into the controversy but pathologists should be aware that differences of opinion exist. The lesions occur usually in the anogenital region, but have been reported in the axilla, the nose, the mucous membranes of the mouth, and the umbilicus.

In addition, it is well to remember that patients with extramammary Paget's disease are prone to develop systemic cancers, usually in neighbouring organs.

H.   UNDIFFERENTIATED CARCINOMA

A malignant epithelial skin tumour that is too poorly differentiated to be placed in any of the groups of carcinomas.

I.   CYSTS

1.   *Keratinous*

(a)   *Pilar cyst* [*trichilemmal, follicular, sebaceous*] (Fig. 55-56)

A lesion lined by rows of squamous-like epithelial cells which degenerate irregularly towards a cystic cavity with swelling of the cells and loss of distinct cell borders.

Rupture of the wall is common and leads to a strong foreign-body giant cell inflammatory reaction. Calcification can be present.

Pilar cysts can reach a considerable size and occur commonly on the scalp and the back but can occur elsewhere. Although usually single, they may occasionally be multiple.

(b)   *Epidermal cyst* (Fig. 57-59)

A cyst lined by stratified squamous epithelium and filled with layers of keratin.

Calcification is occasionally present and rupture of part of the wall may result in a foreign body giant cell inflammatory reaction.

Milia are histologically similar to epidermal cysts but tiny and usually multiple.

Clinically, epidermal cysts are indistinguishable from pilar cysts but the cavity of the pilar cyst contains histologically amorphous material. Proliferation of squamous epithelium may result in what is called a " proliferating cyst " (Fig. 59).

2. *Dermoid cyst* (Fig. 60)

A cyst whose wall contains elements of skin, including a squamous lining, hair follicles, and sebaceous glands.

The lesions are more common on the face in the region of the facial clefts.

3. *Others*

This category includes branchial cleft cysts, bronchogenic cysts, etc.

J. EPITHELIAL TUMOUR-LIKE LESIONS

1. *Seborrhoeic keratosis* (Fig. 61-63)

A lesion characterized by an elevated area of acanthotic epidermis associated with papillomatosis, hyperkeratosis, and invaginations forming horn cysts.

As the tumour grows upwards, the base forms more or less a straight line connecting the level of the normal epidermis on both sides. The tumour is composed of broad interconnecting bands of cells containing the horn cysts. The cells are usually very similar to the basal cells of the epidermis and are consequently called " basaloid ". Squamous cells in varying numbers form the other cellular component. A predominance of one or the other may warrant a distinction between " basal cell type " and " hyperkeratotic " or " acanthotic " type. Hyperpigmentation in the basal layer is quite common and may be present inside the thick epidermal bands. The lesion, which is usually broad-based, may be polypoid. A variety known as the reticulated or adenoid type is also recognized and in this thin bands extend from the epidermis into the corium and show branching and interweaving. These tracts are composed of at least a double row of basaloid cells while horn cysts are usually absent. The different varieties, including the reticulated type, can occur in various combinations.

Irritated lesions may show considerable squamous cell proliferation that simulates a squamous cell carcinoma. In such cases, a strong inflammatory reaction, predominantly of a lymphocytic nature, is present in the stroma.

This extremely common lesion occurs on the trunk, arms and face in middle-aged or elderly people. It is sometimes multiple and can reach a fair size. In characteristic cases the lesions are warty in appearance, brown to nearly black, sharply demarcated, and may look as if " stuck on " to the skin. They are also known as seborrhoeic or senile warts and basal cell papillomas.

2. *Keratoacanthoma* (Fig. 64-65)

> An elevated lesion composed of squamous epithelium with excessive keratin formation filling a central crater.

From the elevated area strands of epidermal cells, often inter-communicating, infiltrate the dermis, commonly reaching close to the subcutaneous tissue. Short upward projections may occur within the central crater. The borders of the crater show lipping towards the centre and in the surrounding epidermis there is acanthosis over a short distance. Para-keratotic cells are commonly present and to a lesser extent atypical cells occur. Particularly in the earlier stages considerable numbers of mitotic figures may be present. The lower border of the epithelium with the corium is often irregular. An inflammatory infiltrate, usually rather dense, is present in the adjoining dermis. In later stages, the breaking up of the cells in the deeper parts of the lesion may provoke a foreign-body giant cell reaction. The histological diagnosis is best made from a low-power examination of a cross-section of the whole lesion. Recurrences and multiple lesions may be found.

This is a rapidly growing lesion, which undergoes spontaneous but slow involution and occurs mainly on the exposed parts of the body (face and hands). Clinically as well as histologically it may simulate squamous cell carcinoma.

3. *Benign squamous keratosis* [*keratotic papilloma*] (Fig. 66-68)

> A lesion with a thick hyperkeratotic layer overlying acanthotic epidermis and usually showing an inflammatory reaction in the dermis.

An occasional horn cyst may be present in the thickened epidermis. Some lesions have pointed, upward projections of the epidermis, which may be so pronounced that the designation " keratotic papilloma " is warranted (Fig. 68). Differentiation from certain forms of actinic (solar) keratosis or seborrhoeic keratosis may be difficult.

4. *Virus lesions*

(*a*) *Verruca vulgaris* (Fig. 69-70)

> A firm, elevated, somewhat papillomatous and hyperkeratotic lesion most commonly occurring on the fingers. A very characteristic feature is the elongation and inbending of the rete ridges at the margins of the lesion. These lesions may be single or multiple and are sometimes quite numerous.

In young lesions, large vacuolated cells, which may contain only a few keratohyaline granules or none at all, can be found in the upper layer of Malpighi and the stratum granulosa amidst granular cells containing heavy clumps of basophilic inclusion material. The nuclei of the vacuolated cells are nearly pyknotic in appearance, basophilic, and surrounded by a clear zone. The plantar wart (verruca plantaris) has a similar histological appearance but is " indented " in the skin and commonly shows much hyperkeratosis and sometimes parakeratosis.

(b) Verruca plana

A lesion in which the epidermis shows considerable acanthosis and hyperkeratosis with numerous large vacuolated cells in the upper Malpighian and granular layers.

As a result of this vacuolar degeneration the overlying stratum corneum shows a basket-weave appearance.

(c) Condyloma acuminatum (Fig. 71)

A verrucous lesion in which the covering epidermis or mucous membrane shows considerable acanthosis with elongation and thickening of the rete ridges. Groups of vacuolated cells in the thickened epithelium are rather characteristic.

A confusing feature can be the presence of large numbers of mitotic figures, but as the arrangement of the squamous cells is orderly and the border with the dermis sharp, malignancy can be ruled out. The underlying stroma is loose, oedematous, and provided with dilated capillaries. A nonspecific chronic inflammation is present, which varies in intensity but is usually rather slight.

These fairly soft verrucous lesions occur in the mucous membranes and skin of the anogenital regions. They can be very numerous and grouped together into cauliflower-like masses.

(d) Molluscum contagiosum (Fig. 72)

A lesion in which the epidermis seems to dip into the underlying dermis forming cup-shaped, closely packed areas containing cells filled with intracytoplasmic inclusion bodies.

The basal layer is free of these bodies. The inclusion bodies change their staining properties from eosinophilic in the deeper layers to basophilic near the surface, while their size increases to such an extent that they ultimately become larger than the original cell they invaded. The nucleus is then compressed at the periphery of the cell.

The lesions present usually as multiple, well circumscribed, small dome-shaped papules.

5. *Hamartomas*

(*a*) *Naevus verrucosus*

This lesion shows villiform or finger-like upward projections with downward elongation of the rete ridges. In addition there is hyperkeratosis and acanthosis.

Keratin can fill up the areas between the villi. Considerable variation can occur in the thickness and apposition of the papillary projections.

(*b*) *Naevus comedonicus*

A lesion in which deep invaginations of the epidermis are filled with keratin and resemble dilated hair follicles.

(*c*) *Others*

Lesions are encountered occasionally which represent malformations of sweat glands, hair follicles or a combination of these structures. As they do not present constant histological features no specific name can be attached. They may occur together with a basal cell carcinoma.

6. *Others*

(*a*) *Acanthosis nigricans*

A papillomatous lesion in which the epidermis shows loose hyperkeratosis, mild acanthosis, and hyperpigmentation. The hyperpigmentation may be slight but is practically always present.

Melanin may be found throughout the whole thickness of the epidermis and small amounts are occasionally released into the dermis.

Although clinically differentiation is made between benign and malignant acanthosis nigricans, occurring respectively in youth and after puberty, histologically the lesions are alike. The term " malignant " refers to the presence of an internal malignancy.

(*b*) *Pseudoepitheliomatous hyperplasia*

A lesion characterized by marked and irregular acanthosis of the epidermis with elongation and widening of rete ridges and with a varying degree of hyperkeratosis, which may be severe. The epidermis may show papillary projections and the underlying dermis usually shows dense chronic inflammation.

The lesions occur locally in an area of infection or disseminated in some systemic diseases (e.g., syphilis, yaws) or poisoning (e.g., bromides). In syphilis and yaws (framboesia) the lesions may be single or multiple (condyloma latum of syphilis, the " yaw " papule of framboesia) and histologically they are fairly characteristic. With appropriate stains the organisms can be identified. In tuberculosis the presence of tubercles in the corium assists in making the correct diagnosis. The presence of micro-abscesses in conjunction with pseudoepitheliomatous hyperplasia must always arouse the suspicion of chromoblastomycosis or other fungal infections (blastomycosis, coccidioidomycosis) and of bromoderma if organisms are absent. Pseudoepitheliomatous hyperplasia is particularly severe in chronic cutaneous amoebiasis and phagedenic ulcers of long standing, leading to the erroneous diagnosis of carcinoma. The development of carcinoma may occur in pseudoepitheliomatous hyperplasia of long standing.

(c) *Isolated dyskeratosis follicularis* [warty dyskeratoma] (Fig. 73-74)

A cup-like invagination of the epidermis containing keratin and para-keratin. The cyst is lined by a layer of epidermal cells covering villi-like projections into the lumen. Acantholytic cells and corps ronds are usually present. Downward growth into the dermis is commonly seen but not to any great depth.

The lesion is an isolated one most commonly occurring on the scalp, face, or neck, but occasionally elsewhere.

(d) *Clear cell acanthoma* (Fig. 75)

A lesion characterized by a sharply defined area in the epidermis in which all the cells, with the exception of the basal layer, are swollen and have a clear appearance. The epidermis is slightly thickened, with mild parakeratosis, and the rete ridges are elongated. In the underlying dermis mild, chronic, nonspecific inflammation is present. The affected epidermal cells are rich in glycogen.

The lesions are slightly elevated, round, flat, and pale-red, and nearly always occur on the legs.

K.   UNCLASSIFIED EPITHELIAL TUMOURS

II. PRECANCEROUS LESIONS AND CONDITIONS

A. ACTINIC KERATOSIS [SOLAR KERATOSIS, SENILE KERATOSIS] (Fig. 76-79)

A lesion in which the epidermis shows considerable hyperkeratosis but usually little or no parakeratosis. The epidermis may be markedly acanthotic and dysplastic epidermal cells may involve part or all of the epidermis. Severe atrophy of the epidermis may occur side by side with acanthosis. The dermis shows extensive basophilic degeneration and contains a nonspecific chronic inflammatory cell infiltrate.

Mild papillomatosis can be present. In some cases atrophy is extreme in the centre of the lesion and the shallow cup-shaped area is filled with keratin. This sometimes forms the base of a cutaneous horn. In the atrophic parts, occasionally comprising most or nearly all of the lesion, the atypical nature of the epidermal cells in the basal layer can lead to tubule-like extensions into the upper dermis and/or clefts just above the basal layer (Fig. 79). In actinic keratosis changes can occur simulating Bowen's disease to a considerable degree.

The lesions frequently present as multiple, rather dry and scaly lesions on parts of the body exposed to the sun in fair-skinned people. Horn-like projections, sometimes several millimetres and in unusual instances even several centimetres in length, can occur in the centre of the atrophic parts of a lesion.

Squamous cell carcinoma and/or basal cell carcinoma may develop in actinic keratosis but this form of squamous cell carcinoma is rarely of high malignancy.

B. RADIATION DERMATOSIS (Fig. 80-81)

Epidermal and dermal alterations caused by ionizing radiation.

The cutaneous effects of ionizing radiation in its chronic form show epidermal changes, which are similar to those found in actinic keratosis but in some areas often grow downward in a peg-like fashion into the dermis. The corium commonly shows mild, chronic, nonspecific inflammation, with considerable degenerative changes, irregular staining, hyalinization, and increase of collagen and reticular fibres. Bizarre fibroblasts are characteristic. The superficial blood vessels are usually dilated and some surrounding oedema may be present. The deeper vessels show obliterative vasculitis and/or thrombosis. In the arterioles or small arteries collections of large cholesterol-containing cells may be present in the media, quite distinct from ordinary atheroma. Of the skin appendages only the sweat glands are still preserved.

C. BOWEN'S DISEASE (Fig. 82-83)

This lesion is a carcinoma-in-situ that involves the whole thickness of the epidermis.

The rete ridges are widened and elongated, with considerable narrowing or even disappearance of the dermal papillae. The epidermal cells have lost their polarity and some may show a clear cytoplasm. Pleomorphism and polychromasia are striking, particularly of the nuclei. Mitotic figures may be present at all levels. Parakeratotic cells may be present and giant nuclei of bizarre forms and clumped nuclei are commonly found. Arsenic ingestion may cause identical lesions, but these are often multiple and may show considerable clear cell change, which should not, however, be regarded as diagnostic.

D. ERYTHROPLASIA OF QUEYRAT

A carcinoma-in-situ with histological changes similar to those seen in Bowen's disease but occurring on the glans penis.

The greater likelihood of infiltration and the lack of proneness to develop systemic cancer warrants their separation from Bowen's disease.

E. INTRAEPIDERMAL EPITHELIOMA OF JADASSOHN (Fig. 84)

A lesion in which interwoven bands of considerably thickened and mildly papillomatous epidermis surround irregular nests of epithelial cells of atypical appearance.

The existence of this lesion as an entity has been challenged because a number of lesions with different intraepidermal changes have all been described under this heading. The group believes that the entity does exist and deserves to be recognized as such.

F. XERODERMA PIGMENTOSUM (Fig. 85)

An irregularly changed epidermis with areas of mild hyperkeratosis, acanthosis, atrophy or proliferation of rete ridges, and focal hyperpigmentation of the basal layer with release of melanin into the dermis, which usually shows rather severe chronic inflammation.

The condition is a hypersensitivity of the skin to sunlight, which is determined by a recessive gene and leads to the development of multiple or successive malignancies (basal cell carcinoma, squamous cell carcinoma, and/or malignant melanoma).

G. Others

A large variety of etiological agents are commonly connected with precancerous changes. That arsenic may act in this way has already been mentioned under Bowen's disease, but tar and oil dermatoses, thermal and chemical injuries, chronic sinuses, and phagedenic ulcers can also lead to precancerous changes. In addition, precancerous changes are occasionally observed in scarred areas of the skin.

III.   TUMOURS AND LESIONS OF THE MELANOGENIC SYSTEM

A.   Benign (naevus)

Lesions arising from melanocytes of the epidermis or dermis and occurring as brown spots of varying size and depth of colour on any part of the skin.

They can be flat, slightly elevated, smooth, or warty in appearance. They can be present at early infancy, but commonly increase in numbers around puberty. Occasionally they occur as huge lesions at birth and are then known as giant pigmented naevi. Histologically many varieties are recognized.

1.   *Junctional naevus* (Fig. 86)

In this lesion nests of naevus cells are found at the epidermal–dermal junction.

The naevus cells are commonly located at the tips of the rete ridges and the basal layer between these areas is normal or may contain a slightly increased number of melanocytes. The remaining epidermis is normal.

2.   *Compound naevus* (Fig. 87)

A lesion in which, in addition to naevus cells at the epidermal–dermal junction as described under 1, there are nests of naevus cells in the dermis to a varying depth.

The lesions are commonly papillary in appearance and may contain hair.

3.   *Intradermal naevus* (Fig. 88-89)

A lesion in which naevus cells are virtually limited to the dermis, although a few naevus cells are nearly always found at the epidermal–dermal junction.

Pure dermal naevi are extremely rare. Multinucleated naevus cells are common.

4. *Epithelioid and/or spindle cell naevus [juvenile melanoma]* (Fig. 90-92)

A compound naevus that occasionally shows considerable junction changes, sometimes with much acanthosis and subepidermal oedema. Melanin pigment is usually minimal or absent. The cells are elongated and/or more rounded and epithelioid in appearance, but both types may occur in the same tumour.

Mitotic figures are sometimes absent but on occasion are quite numerous. The spindle-shaped cells are often arranged in fascicles perpendicular to the epidermis. In the epithelioid type a characteristic feature is the presence of mononucleated and multinucleated giant cells of irregular shape. The multinucleated giant cells may show an irregular distribution of nuclei, which are sometimes either clumped or arranged at the periphery, simulating somewhat the Touton type of giant cell. This naevus is frequently confused with malignant melanoma on histological grounds.

It is a benign dome-shaped lesion commonly occurring on the face but also elsewhere and most often seen in children.

5. *Balloon cell naevus* (Fig. 93-94)

A naevus in which many of the cells have clear cytoplasm and are commonly enlarged up to ten times the size of normal naevus cells. The nuclei are uniform.

The balloon cells may be irregularly distributed and may be present in small amounts, or they may occupy large areas. Balloon cell naevi have sometimes been mistaken histologically for xanthoma.

6. *Halo naevus* (Fig. 95-96)

A naevus surrounded by a depigmented zone, the halo. Naevus cell nests can usually still be recognized in the upper zone of the dermis but invaded and partly replaced by a dense infiltrate of lymphocyte-like cells amongst which larger cells of a more histiocytic appearance occur.

Melanin is scattered throughout the infiltrate. In darker-skinned people the surrounding epidermis shows depigmentation in conformity with the clinical appearance.

7. *Giant pigmented naevus* (Fig. 97-99)

A naevus showing both a superficial and a deep pattern; the superficial pattern is that of a compound or intradermal naevus and the deep pattern shows fusiform and spindle-shaped cells loosely arranged in sheets or nodules. Typically, the tissue of the deep pattern extends into the subcutaneous tissue.

Neuroid structures may be seen. Melanin pigment is most pronounced in the epidermis and upper dermis.

The giant pigmented naevus is congenital, often large, and may affect the scalp, trunk, and extremities. Satellite naevi are common. It is usually darkly pigmented, hairy, and may be nodular. It is sometimes associated with central nervous system melanocytosis. Malignant melanoma develops in about one-third of the patients.

8. *Fibrous papule of the nose* [*involuting naevus*]

A dome-shaped or papular elevation of the skin composed of fibrous tissue within which multinucleated giant cells are often scattered. Melanocytes tend to be numerous at the dermal–epidermal junction and occasionally nests of naevus cells are present. Blood vessels are ectatic.

Clinically the fibrous papule has a pigmented or angiomatous appearance and is usually located on the nose near the ali nasa. The lesion probably represents a naevus undergoing fibrosis.

9. *Blue naevus* (Fig. 100-101)

A naevus located in the dermis and composed of elongated melanocytes with spindly, sometimes dendritic-looking projections.

The cells are commonly packed in groups and these may extend into the subcutaneous fat. Generally these pigmented cells lie parallel to the epidermis. The dendritic projections become particularly clear in silver stains.

The blue naevus is a sharply circumscribed nodular lesion usually measuring no more than 15 mm in diameter and of bluish to blue-grey colour. It occurs most commonly on the face or around the forearms and hands. For minor differences between blue naevus and the naevus of Ota and the naevus of Ito specialized textbooks or relevant articles should be consulted.

10. *Cellular blue naevus* (Fig. 102-104)

> A blue naevus in which the melanocytic cells are much more numerous and closely packed and may form intertwining bundles having some similarity to nerve bundles.

This type of naevus has a striking appearance as the cells are not only of the elongated dendritic type but also more fusiform, larger, and sometimes rounded. The nuclei also vary in size and the cytoplasm may contain only little pigment as a result of which the cells show up with pale, abundant cytoplasm. The melanin distribution is highly irregular. The lesion may extend into the subcutaneous fat, sometimes to a considerable depth. On occasion the lesion may be large (several centimetres in diameter), deep black in colour, and show an extremely variegated picture. Malignant melanoma arising in a cellular blue naevus is extremely rare and should be diagnosed only when there is unequivocal evidence. The impossibility of finding mitoses, the presence of the dendritic type of cell in some areas of the lesion, and the absence of necrosis all favour a benign lesion.

Rarely a cellular blue naevus metastasizes, but usually only to the regional lymph nodes where the histological picture is similar to that seen in the skin. The prognosis is usually excellent.

B. PRECANCEROUS

1. *Precancerous melanosis including Hutchinson's melanotic freckle* (Fig. 105-108)

> An accumulation of mainly abnormal melanocytes along the lower border of the epidermis and occasionally accompanied by similar cells throughout the whole thickness of the epidermis; the outer layer of the hair follicles may also be involved.

Histologically the picture varies with the age of the lesion and from one lesion to the other or in one and the same lesion from one area to another. In the first-formed parts of the lesions, before the melanotic freckle is fully developed, dysplastic melanocytic cells may be present throughout the epidermis; they often contain melanin and an occasional mitotic figure. This picture can also be found in the periphery of a fully developed or enlarging lesion. In the fully developed lesion the rete ridges have flattened out and the epidermis may be atrophic. The nuclei of the melanocytes may be atypical or nearly pyknotic and occasionally mitotic figures can be found, but in other cases the melanocytes may have a swollen balloon-shaped aspect with either eosinophilic or clear cytoplasm. Relatively small, clear melanocytes and/or the larger forms may be scattered through the whole thickness of the epidermis. In the basal layer the cells may take on a more elongated, spindly form and not uncommonly it may be difficult to decide if early invasion into the dermal papillae has taken place.

In parts of the skin exposed to the sun, particularly in the classical Hutchinson's melanotic freckle arising in the malar region of the face, there is basophilic degeneration of the corium (elastosis) and a scattered non-specific inflammatory infiltrate of varying density is present in the upper layer of the corium.

Clinically these are usually pigmented lesions that enlarge slowly and irregularly and are of variegated colour; they arise not only in the malar region of the face in middle-aged and elderly people (the classical Hutchinson's melanotic freckle), but occasionally start much earlier in life or in a different site. Not uncommonly, lesions of the latter kind also develop more quickly to a malignant form.

C. MALIGNANT

1. *Malignant melanoma* (Fig. 109-119)

A highly malignant tumour consisting of abnormal melanocytes of a cuboidal, polygonal, or spindle shape, which are pigmented to a varying degree.

Histologically malignant melanoma nearly always arises in the epidermodermal junction, and it is sometimes associated with the presence of a pre-existing naevus.

Histologically abnormal melanocytes of a cuboidal, polygonal, or spindle shape infiltrate downwards into the dermis and occasionally upwards into the epidermis, ultimately leading to ulceration. The cuboidal melanocytic cells usually show a well-defined cytoplasmic border, with an eosinophilic or more commonly a characteristically amphophilic cytoplasm, and a fairly large, round nucleus with a distinct, large, round nucleolus. Multinucleated giant cells may occur. In the spindle-cell variety the cells are elongated and the cell types in both cellular varieties may form compact masses. The melanin pigmentation not only varies considerably from tumour to tumour but also within any given tumour in different areas. Occasionally tumours contain hardly any detectable pigment or none at all. It is advisable in such cases to apply an appropriate melanin stain (e.g., Fontana) to detect the small amounts of melanin that may be present. The number of mitotic figures varies considerably from tumour to tumour and within one and the same tumour. They can be quite numerous or extremely sparse. Tumours do occur containing mixtures of cuboidal epithelioid and spindle-shaped cells, but the cuboidal and polygonal forms are the most common. The rare occurrence of a malignant melanoma entirely composed of balloon cells has been observed. In the surrounding stroma, a nonspecific, chronic inflammatory infiltrate of varying density is commonly present. Fixation artefacts may sometimes give rise to small slit-like spaces around seemingly isolated cell groups or infiltrating strands, but these should not be mistaken for infiltrations into the lymphatics. Such infiltrations can be accepted unequivocally only when the spaces are lined by clearly distinguishable endothelium. Partial regression occurs not infrequently and in such cases a dense inflammatory infiltrate seems to break up and destroy parts of the tumour (Fig. 118-119). In rare instances, complete regression can be observed, leaving histologically only an irregular layer of melanin in the corium.

The tumours are flat, slightly elevated, dome-shaped, or polypoidal in appearance and affect all ages, but they are very rare before puberty. They can arise in any part of the skin including the nailbeds (melanotic whitlow). Malignant melanoma on the sole of the foot is rare, except in pigmented people who go barefoot. Malignant melanomas arising in the eye and those arising occasionally in other sites (oral cavity, nose, bronchus, meninges, etc.) form a separate group and are not discussed here. Melanomas occur not infrequently in patients afflicted with xeroderma pigmentosum and in pigmented people in conjunction with partial albinism, or in areas with local depigmentation. The presence or absence of preceding skin changes as mentioned should be noted.

2. *Malignant melanoma arising in precancerous melanosis, including Hutchinson's melanotic freckle* (Fig. 120)

The occurrence of melanoma is determined by the presence of atypical melanocytic cells invading the corium. In many instances but not always the invading cells are spindle-shaped.

Some authors recognize a category of melanoma in which there is seeming lateral spread and in which histologically there are collections of cells with clear cytoplasm that have been called " pagetoid " because of their resemblance to Paget cells. This pattern has been designated by those authors as " superficial spreading melanoma " and is distinguished from the nodular pattern. In our experience this distinction is not always easily or readily accomplished. Additionally, it is sometimes difficult to distinguish histologically between the epidermal manifestations of so-called superficial spreading melanoma and precancerous melanosis wherever it occurs, since different histologic patterns may be present. Wide sampling of these lesions is advisable to detect invasion when obvious invasion has not yet taken place. The melanoma arising in a Hutchinson's melanotic freckle has generally a much better prognosis than one arising in a precancerous melanosis at a different site.

3. *Malignant melanoma arising in a blue naevus* (Fig. 121)

   The melanomas arising in cellular blue naevi have a far better prognosis than others, even when secondary manifestations appear in lymph nodes.

4. *Malignant melanoma arising in a giant pigmented naevus* (Fig. 97)

   This melanoma arises at an earlier age than other melanomas and usually in the dermal part of the lesion.

D.   Non-tumorous Pigmented Lesions

1. *Mongolian spot*

   This lesion is characterized by the presence of fusiform dendritic dopa-positive melanin-containing cells, particularly in the lower half of the dermis and most commonly in the lumbosacral region.

   Although most frequently found in Mongolian people, it also occurs occasionally in other ethnic races and at sites other than the back, and multiple spots have been observed.

2. *Lentigo* (Fig. 122)

   This lesion is formed by elongations of the rete ridges with an increased melanin content as well as increased numbers of melanocytes.

   Clinically, juvenile and senile forms of lentigo are distinguished depending on the time of life at which they occur. In the senile form flattening of the rete ridges may occur and differentiation from precancerous melanosis may be difficult.

   When lentigo occurs on parts exposed to the sun, basophilic degeneration of the dermis is usually evident.

3. *Ephelis* (Fig. 123)

   A lesion characterized by increased melanin pigmentation in a localized area of an essentially normal epidermis. The number of melanocytes is not normally increased and is commonly decreased.

IV. SOFT TISSUE TUMOURS AND TUMOUR-LIKE LESIONS

Definitions and explanatory notes for this group of tumours are, in general, limited to those entities peculiar to the skin. For notes on the other items included in this classification, reference should be made to *Histological Typing of Soft Tissue Tumours* (IHCT No. 3, see p. 6).

A. TUMOURS OF FIBROUS TISSUE

1. *Benign*

    (a) *Fibroma*

    (b) *Dermatofibroma [histiocytoma, sclerosing haemangioma]* (Fig. 124-125)

    An ill-defined lesion showing a mixture of fibroblastic and histiocytic cells with varying amounts of collagen and thin-walled blood vessels.

    Siderophages and lipid-containing macrophages are frequently present and may give the lesion a yellowish to deep brown colour. Small multinucleated giant cells (Touton giant cells) are sometimes encountered.

2. *Malignant*

    (a) *Dermatofibrosarcoma protuberans* (Fig. 126-127)

    A cellular tumour composed of small, uniform, fibrocytic cells, often arranged in a cartwheel pattern.

    This tumour usually forms a protruding nodular or multinodular mass by infiltration of the entire dermis and the subcutaneous fat. The tumour has a tendency to recur locally after simple excision. Cases with metastases have been recorded.

    (b) *Fibrosarcoma*

3. *Tumour-like lesions*

    (a) *Cutaneous fibrous polyp [skin tag]* (Fig. 128)

    This consists of a fibrous core of varying density covered by an essentially normal epidermis.

    The growth may be present at birth and commonly occurs on the head as a soft, slightly wrinkled, polypoid lesion.

(b) *Hyperplastic scar* (Fig. 129)

(c) *Keloid* (Fig. 130-131)

A superficial nodular growth formed by small fibrocytic and/or fibroblastic cells in various numbers lying between characteristic, well-
defined, broad bands of homogeneous acidophilic collagen.

The lesion usually follows some form of injury to the skin and is found
mainly in heavily pigmented people. Unlike hypertrophic scars, which
do not show the characteristic thick glassy collagen bundles, keloid tends
to recur.

(d) *Nodular fasciitis*

B. TUMOURS OF FAT TISSUE

1. *Benign*

(a) *Lipoma*

(b) *Angiolipoma*

(c) *Hibernoma*

2. *Malignant*

(a) *Liposarcoma*

C. TUMOURS OF MUSCLE

1. *Benign*

(a) *Leiomyoma* (Fig. 132-133)

2. *Malignant*

(a) *Leiomyosarcoma* (Fig. 134-135)

D. TUMOURS OF BLOOD VESSELS

1. *Benign*

(a) *Haemangioma of granulation tissue type* [*granuloma pyogenicum*] (Fig. 136)

A benign, solitary, raised lesion of the skin and mucous membranes having the microscopic appearance of a lobulated capillary haemangioma or richly vascular granulation tissue.

Secondary features, such as surface ulceration, chronic inflammation, and fibrosis are common.

(b) *Capillary haemangioma* [*juvenile haemangioma*]

(c) *Cavernous haemangioma*

(d) *Verrucous keratotic haemangioma* (Fig. 137-138)

A lesion in which the epidermis shows verruciform projections with dilated capillaries in close apposition to the basal layer and simulating angiokeratoma, but with vascular changes extending into the underlying dermis and subcutis, usually in the form of a capillary angioma.

An erroneous diagnosis of angiokeratoma would lead to inadequate treatment.

(e) *Glomus tumour group*

(i) glomus tumour (Fig. 139)

(ii) glomangioma

(iii) angiomyoma (Fig. 140)

(f) *Angiokeratoma*

This lesion is characterized by a slightly hyperkeratotic epidermis with some acanthosis overlying widely dilated blood spaces lined by a single endothelial layer. The epidermis extends and sometimes appears to surround these blood spaces. The whole lesion can be warty or even polypoid.

(i) Mibelli and Fordyce types (Fig. 141-142)

The difference between the two types lies in the distribution of the lesions, which are histologically identical. In the Mibelli type there are multiple, slightly warty, reddish nodules on the dorsum of the fingers and toes. In the Fordyce type they are single or multiple and commonly occur on the scrotum.

(ii) Fabry type [angiokeratoma corporis diffusum] (Fig. 143-144)

A lesion very similar to other angiokeratomas but without the hyperkeratosis and with lipid deposition in the endothelial and muscle
cells of small blood vessels in the skin.

This is a systemic and ultimately fatal lipid storage disease in which
large amounts of glycolipids are stored in the endothelial cells and smooth
muscle cells of the blood vessels and skin; it also affects the renal glomeruli
and the myocardium. The multiple small skin lesions appear usually around
puberty.

(g) *Others* (Fig. 145)

2. *Malignant*

(a) *Angiosarcoma [malignant haemangioendothelioma]* (Fig. 146)

(b) *Kaposi's sarcoma [multiple idiopathic haemorrhagic sarcoma]*
(Fig. 147-149)

A lesion made up of irregular vascular channels and spaces, formed
and surrounded by slender spindle-shaped cells with prominent,
deeply-staining nuclei, superficially resembling leiomyoblasts.

The lesions are usually multiple and may occur in the skin as well as
in the viscera. Haemosiderin pigment is frequently found. The histogenesis
is obscure. The tumour is occasionally associated with malignant lymphoma.

In the early stages the lesion shows a reaction of the vascular granulation type with many dilated and poorly formed capillaries and with big
endothelial cells protruding into the lumen and surrounded by oedematous
connective tissue containing a nonspecific infiltrate composed of lympho-
cytes, plasma cells, and occasional histiocytic cells. The presence of small
extravasations of erythrocytes and of haemosiderin pigment are common.
In the established lesion there is a characteristic proliferation of elongated
cells in between which are rows of erythrocytes forming a vascular slit
pattern. In the periphery of such lesions increased numbers of dilated
blood vessels are found, giving an angiomatous appearance.

The disease is characterized by multiple papular or plaque-like lesions
on the distal part of the extremities, most commonly on the lower legs and
feet. Single lesions occur occasionally, and visceral manifestations have
been noted.

3. *Tumour-like lesions*

(a) *Reactive blood vessel hyperplasia*

E. TUMOURS OF LYMPH VESSELS

1. *Benign*[1]

2. *Malignant*[1]

F. TUMOURS OF THE PERIPHERAL NERVES

1. *Benign*[1]

Neurofibromatosis [von Recklinghausen's disease] is a condition inherited through an autosomal dominant in which a varying but commonly large number of peripheral nerve tumours of all varieties occur in the skin. Malignant change is a well-known complication, but is usually confined to a single tumour.

2. *Malignant*[1]

3. *Tumour-like lesions*

(*a*) *Traumatic neuroma*

(*b*) *Nasal glioma* (Fig. 150)

A congenital lesion, at the base of the nose, in which nerve tissue, practically always glial in nature, extends into the dermis.

Sometimes associated with inadequate closure of the frontal bones, the lesion is probably initially a meningoencephalocele, becoming separated later.

(*c*) *Cutaneous meningioma* (Fig. 151)

A lesion consisting of meningothelial cells with psammoma bodies and so-called collagen bodies in the dermis and subcutis.

A primary form occurs in children and most likely represents a developmental defect. A secondary form that occurs in older persons follows the distribution of the cranial nerves and is more destructive, invading muscle and bone and leading to ulceration of the overlying epidermis.

(*d*) *Others*

---

[1] For the subgroups of these categories, see the Classification, pp. 21 and 22.

G. TUMOUR-LIKE XANTHOMATOUS LESIONS

1. *Xanthoma* (Fig. 152)

> A benign growth made up chiefly of xanthoma cells (lipid-carrying
> histiocytes), occasional Touton-type giant cells, and varying amounts
> of fibrous connective tissue.

The lesion may be solitary or multiple and is often associated with
high levels of serum cholesterol and phospholipid (hypercholesteraemic
xanthomatosis).

2. *Fibroxanthoma*

3. *Atypical fibroxanthoma* (Fig. 153-155)

> An ulceronodular lesion containing multinucleated giant cells of bizarre
> appearance and atypical mitotic figures among fibrous and xantho-
> matous cells.

The tumour characteristically occurs on the exposed areas of the skin
(the head and neck) in older people, but an apparent variant occurs on
covered areas of the body in younger people. Occasionally the lesion extends
into the subcutaneous fat. The lesion follows a benign course in nearly
all instances.

4. *Juvenile xanthogranuloma* [*naevo-xanthoendothelioma*] (Fig. 156-157)

5. *Reticulohistiocytic granuloma* [*reticulohistiocytoma*] (Fig. 158-159)

> A lesion consisting of a mass of closely packed, large, globular his-
> tiocytic cells with eosinophilic cytoplasm, which is sometimes
> somewhat glassy in appearance. The nuclei are vesicular, with a
> small pronounced nucleolus, and are occasionally indented.

With appropriate fat stains faint staining of the cytoplasm is obtained.
Giant cells and multinucleated cells can occur. The stroma commonly
shows nonspecific inflammation.

It is a nodular solitary lesion occurring in the skin. The cut surface
commonly has a yellowish appearance. Multiple lesions sometimes occur
in association with arthritis. The relationship of this group to the single
lesions is unknown.

H. Miscellaneous tumours and tumour-like lesions

1. *Granular cell tumour*

2. *Osteoma cutis* (Fig. 160)

An ossifying lesion in the dermis.

This lesion can occur as a reactive phenomenon and is not uncommonly found as such in association with other lesions, or it may occur as a real tumour in the dermis extending into the subcutis.

3. *Chondroma cutis* (Fig. 161)

4. *Myxoma*

5. *Cutaneous focal mucinosis*

A localized area in the corium in which the collagen is partially replaced by pale-staining myxomatous fibroblastic stroma.

Clinically the lesion appears as a solitary, asymptomatic, flesh-coloured nodule.

6. *Cutaneous myxoid cyst* (Fig. 162)

A cystic area of the fingers or toes in which the collagen is replaced by mucin. The lesion has also been called synovial cyst and ganglion.

7. *Fibrous hamartoma of infancy* (Fig. 163)

A lesion composed of well-defined bundles of dense fibrocollagenous tissue, which traverse, mix with and surround loose-textured cellular areas of immature appearance and intermingle with mature fat.

They extend from the lower part of the dermis into the subcutaneous tissue and can reach a large size. These tumours occur most frequently in the axilla, shoulder, and upper-arm regions. Boys are more commonly affected than girls. The tumours nearly always appear within the first two years of life and can be present at birth.

8. *Recurring digital fibroma* (Fig. 164)

> A fibroblastic proliferation extending from a slightly acanthotic epider-
> mis to deep into the subcutaneous fat and in which some of the
> fibroblasts contain small, round, or ovoid intracytoplasmic inclusion
> bodies ranging from 3 to 10 microns in diameter.

The tumours occur on the toes and fingers of young children and can
be present at birth. They are slow growing and have a tendency to recur
after surgical removal.

9. *Pseudosarcoma* (Fig. 165-166)

> An ulcerating lesion with a variegated histological picture composed
> of interlacing bundles of elongated cells with numerous mitoses,
> occasionally in the presence of giant cells and partially oedematous
> stroma, which may contain scattered inflammatory cells.

The lesion extends deep into the dermis and occasionally into the
subcutis. The features are reminiscent of leiomyosarcoma in some cases,
in others they simulate cutaneous nodular fasciitis and occasionally seem
to belong to the atypical fibroxanthoma group. Like the latter tumours,
the lesions are found mainly on the face in elderly people and are benign,
notwithstanding the ominous histological features.

10. *Rheumatoid nodule*

11. *Pseudorheumatoid nodule* [*deep granuloma annulare*]

12. *Tumoral calcinosis* (Fig. 167)

> A lesion in which fibrous strands surround areas of proteinaceous
> material containing irregular calcium deposits. Reactive foreign
> body giant cells are usually numerous.

The lesions can become large and can be multiple. They are most
commonly found in relation to joints.

13. *Others*

V. TUMOURS AND TUMOUR-LIKE CONDITIONS OF THE HAEMATOPOIETIC AND LYMPHOID TISSUES

A. MYCOSIS FUNGOIDES (Fig. 168-171)

A condition characterized histologically by a polymorphous cellular dermal infiltrate with numerous atypical lymphoid cells and sometimes multinucleated cells with clumped nuclei.

Intraepidermal clusters of atypical lymphoid cells form Pautrier " microabscesses " but these are not always present. In thin sections the nuclei of the lymphoid cells have a cerebriform (hyperconvoluted) appearance.
Clinically, mycosis fungoides is often manifested by erythematous (premycotic), plaque-like, and tumour stages, and sometimes simultaneous occurrence of all three stages. The histological picture of mycosis fungoides in the premycotic stage is seldom distinctive. In the tumour stage the infiltrate becomes increasingly monomorphous and the histological picture may resemble that of a lymphosarcoma or reticulum cell sarcoma.

B. URTICARIA PIGMENTOSA [MASTOCYTOMA] (Fig. 172-173)

A heavy infiltration of mast cells throughout the dermis with mainly oval or spindle-shaped nuclei.

The cytoplasm contains metachromatic granules that can be made visible with appropriate stains (methylene blue, toluidine blue, Leder, Giemsa). The lesions are usually multiple, but occasionally single lesions occur. Rarely there is systemic involvement.

C. LEUKAEMIAS AND LYMPHOMAS

The classification of these tumours will be included in *Histological and Cytological Typing of Neoplastic Diseases of Haematopoietic and Lymphoid Tissues*, which is at present in preparation by WHO.

D. REACTIVE LYMPHOID HYPERPLASIA (Fig. 174-175)

A lesion in which dense lymphocytic infiltrations occur in the dermis.

The centre of the infiltrations may show follicular structures with germinal centres. In most instances, an additional polymorphous cellular infiltrate is present. Occasionally, remnants of the causative factor can be found (e.g., proboscis of an arthropod). Usually the cause is not known.

E. BENIGN LYMPHOCYTOMA CUTIS (Fig. 176)

> A dense infiltration of lymphocytes and histiocytes in the dermis, usually separated from the epidermis by a thin layer of normal collagen fibres.

The two cell types can be mixed or arranged in distinct follicles. Occasionally some plasma cells and/or eosinophils may be present. A differential diagnosis between this condition and reactive lymphoid hyperplasia may be impossible and differentiation from lymphosarcoma can be very difficult.

F. BENIGN LYMPHOCYTIC INFILTRATE OF JESSNER

> Large, reasonably well demarcated areas composed almost entirely of lymphocytes in the dermis, concentrated preferentially around blood vessels and skin appendages.

The lesions occur on the face and commonly also on the back. There is still no agreement as to whether the lesion represents a separate entity or is to be considered a variant of chronic discoid lupus erythematosus.

G. HISTIOCYTOSIS X

H. EOSINOPHILIC GRANULOMA

VI.   METASTATIC TUMOURS

VII.   UNCLASSIFIED TUMOURS

Unless otherwise stated, all the preparations shown in the photomicrographs reproduced on the following pages were stained with haematoxylin-eosin.

INDEX*

---

* The names printed in heavy type are the terms used in the Classification.

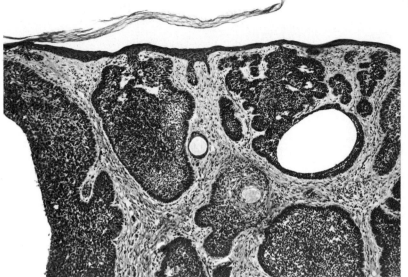

× 80

Fig. 1. Basal cell carcinoma
Solid and cystic areas

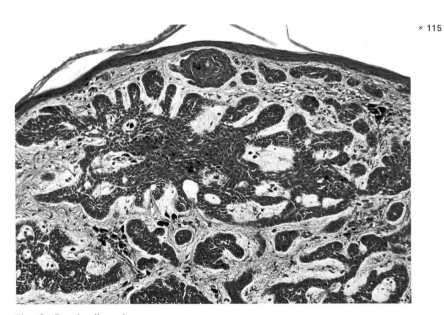

× 115

Fig. 2. Basal cell carcinoma
Pigmented

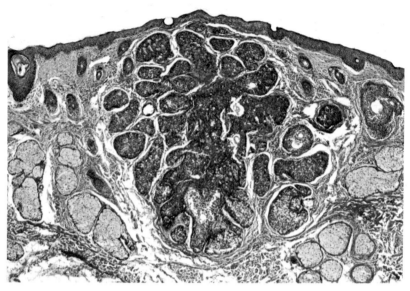

Fig. 3. Basal cell carcinoma
Sebaceous differentiation

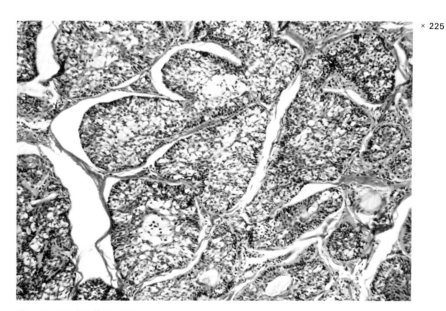

Fig. 4. Basal cell carcinoma
Sebaceous differentiation

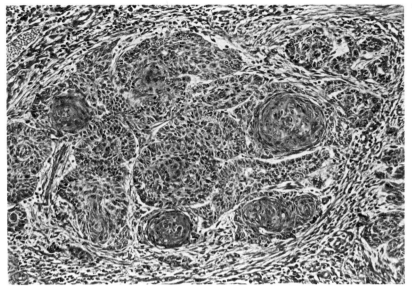

× 115

Fig. 5. Basal cell carcinoma
Foci of keratinization

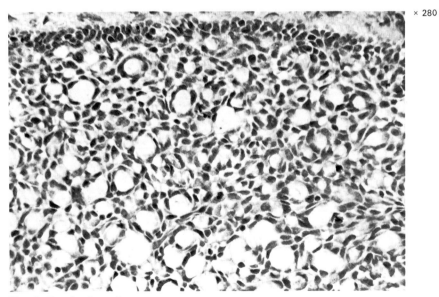

× 280

Fig. 6. Basal cell carcinoma
Microcystic adenoid pattern

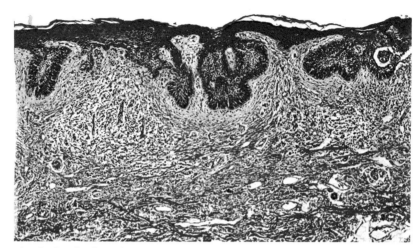

Fig. 7. Basal cell carcinoma, superficial multicentric type

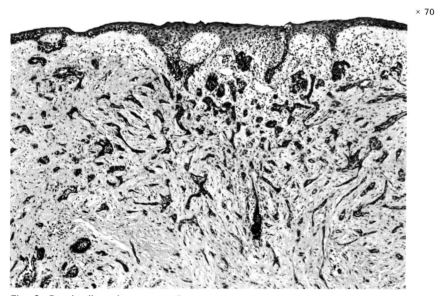

Fig. 8. Basal cell carcinoma, morphoea type

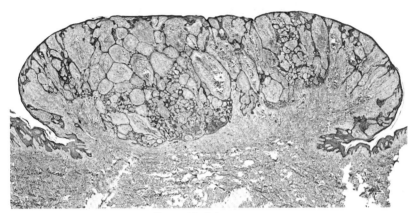

Fig. 9. Basal cell carcinoma, fibroepithelial type

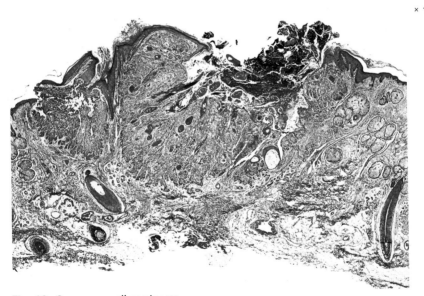

Fig. 10. Squamous cell carcinoma

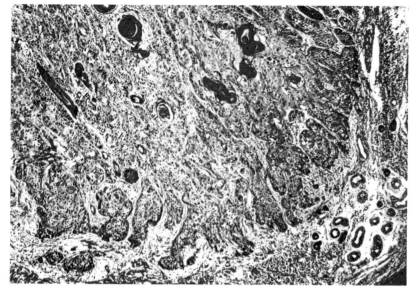

× 35

Fig. 11. Squamous cell carcinoma
Invasion of corium

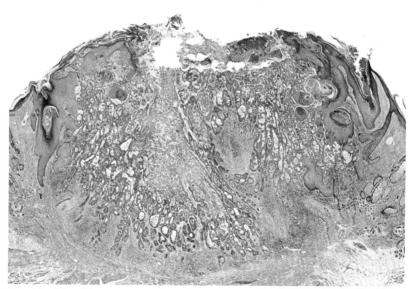

× 11

Fig. 12. Adenoid squamous cell carcinoma

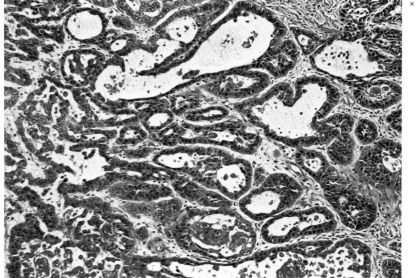

× 80

Fig. 13. Adenoid squamous cell carcinoma

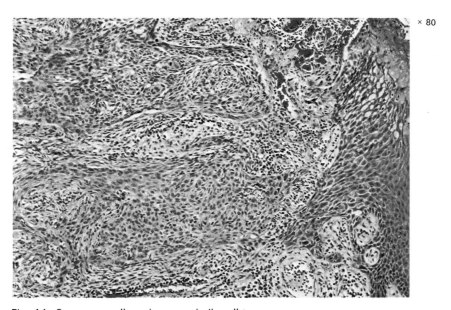

× 80

Fig. 14. Squamous cell carcinoma, spindle cell type

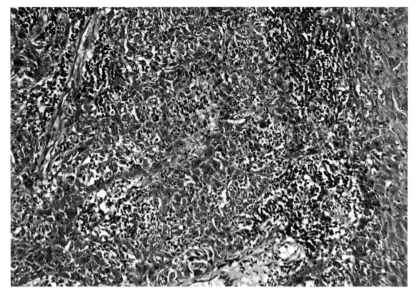

× 115

Fig. 15. Squamous cell carcinoma
Poorly differentiated. Well differentiated squamous epithelium on the right

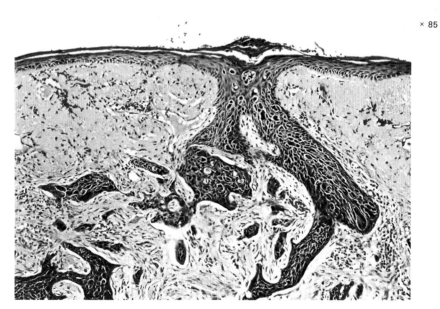

× 85

Fig. 16. Metatypical carcinoma

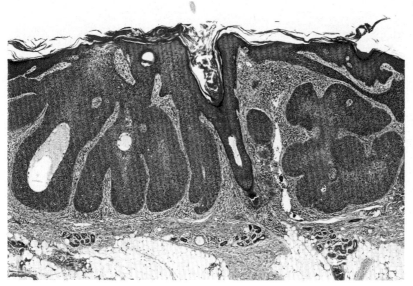

Fig. 17. Metatypical carcinoma
Growth pattern simulating basal cell carcinoma

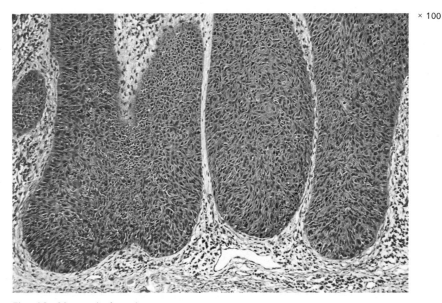

Fig. 18. Metatypical carcinoma
Growth pattern simulating basal cell carcinoma

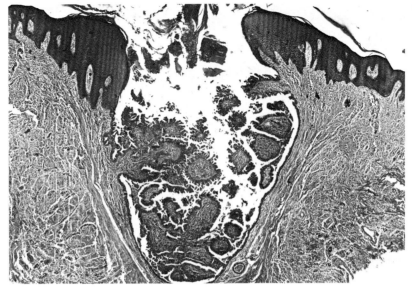

Fig. 19. Papillary syringadenoma

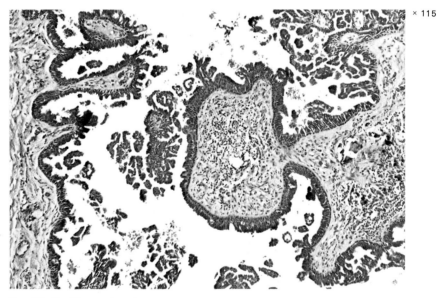

Fig. 20. Papillary syringadenoma
Double layer of epithelium. Plasma cells in stroma. Haemosiderin present

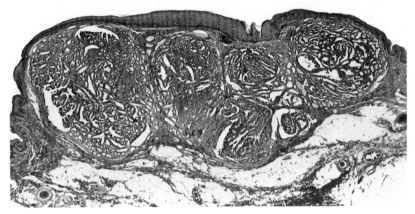

Fig. 21. Papillary hidradenoma
Subepidermal location. Lace-like pattern

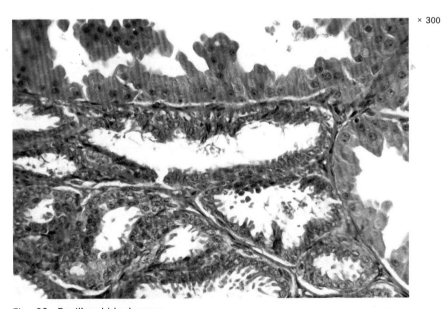

Fig. 22. Papillary hidradenoma
Acidophil cells and " decapitation " cells

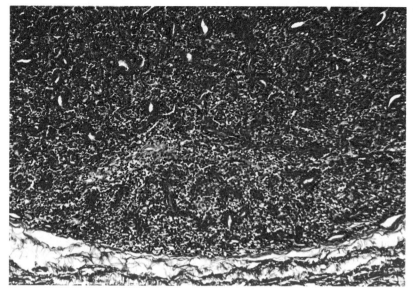

Fig. 23. Eccrine spiradenoma
Well-defined margin

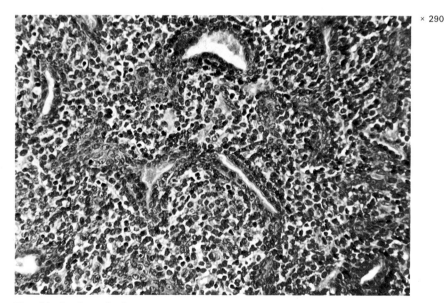

Fig. 24. Eccrine spiradenoma
Pale and dark cells and glandular pattern

× 3.6

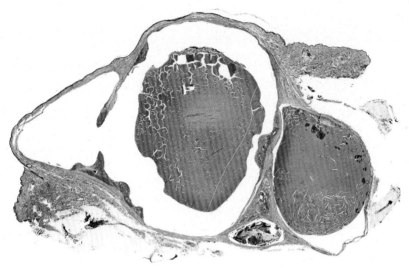

Fig. 25. Eccrine acrospiroma
Predominantly cystic

× 13

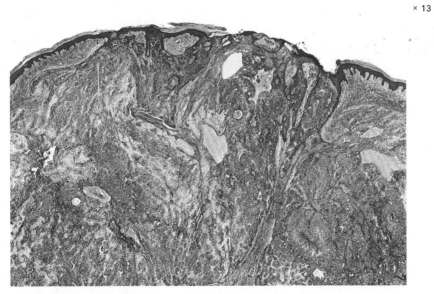

Fig. 26. Eccrine acrospiroma
Predominantly solid

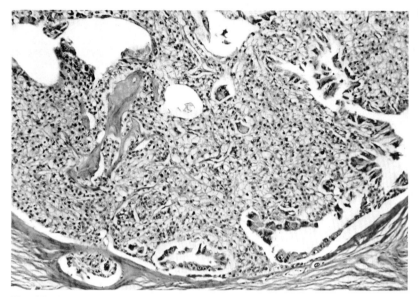

Fig. 27. Eccrine acrospiroma
Clear cells. Small cysts

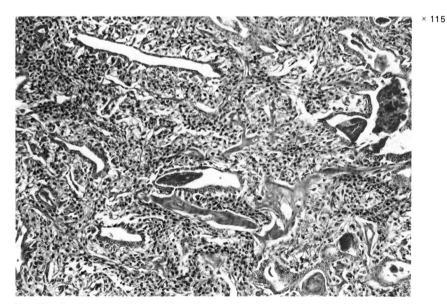

Fig. 28. Eccrine acrospiroma
Clear cells and acidophilic cells. Duct-like structures

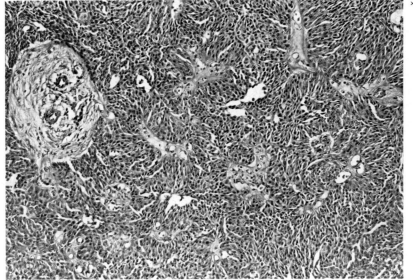

× 115

Fig. 29. Eccrine acrospiroma
Elongated acidophilic cells. Rosette-like pattern

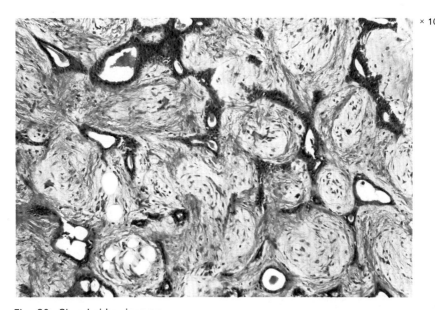

× 100

Fig. 30. Chondroid syringoma

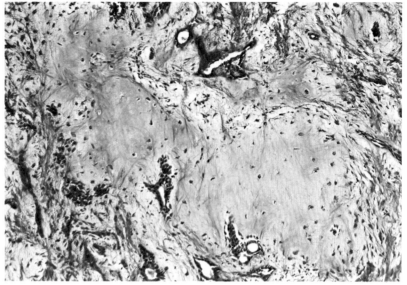

Fig. 31. Chondroid syringoma

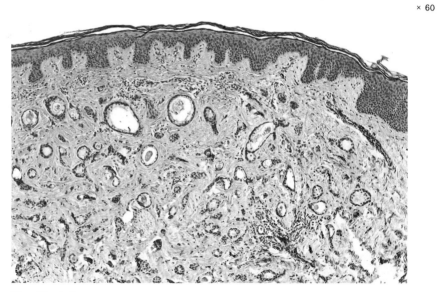

Fig. 32. Syringoma

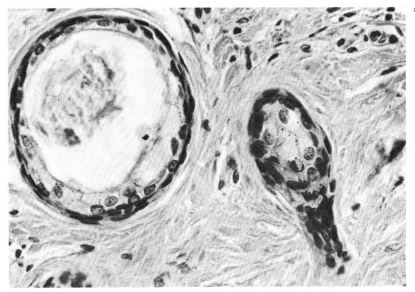

Fig. 33. Syringoma

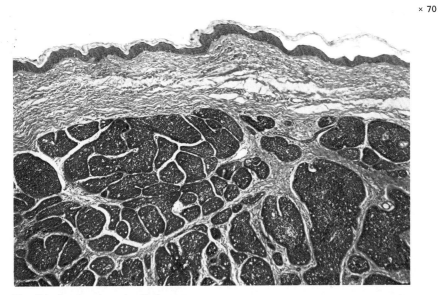

Fig. 34. Eccrine dermal cylindroma

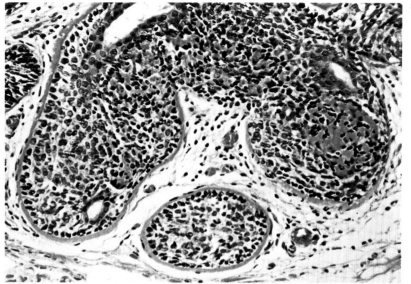

× 250

Fig. 35. Eccrine dermal cylindroma
  Hyalin around and within epithelial cords

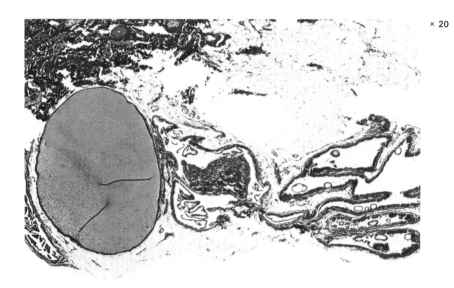

× 20

Fig. 36. Hidrocystoma

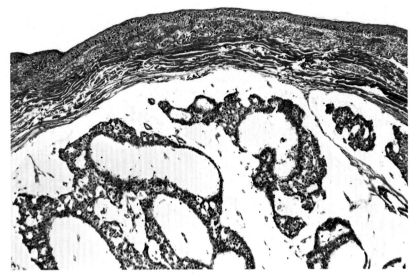

Fig. 37. Mucinous adenocarcinoma

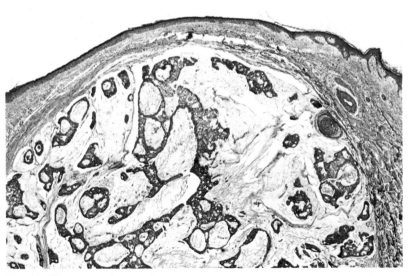

Fig. 38. Mucinous adenocarcinoma
Same tumour as Fig. 37. Movat's pentachrome stain

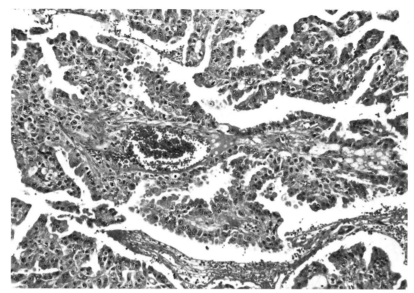

Fig. 39. Sweat gland carcinoma
Papillary pattern. Apocrine-type cells

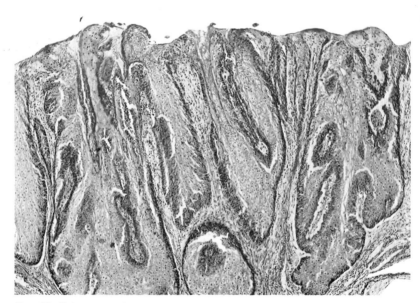

Fig. 40. Sebaceous adenoma

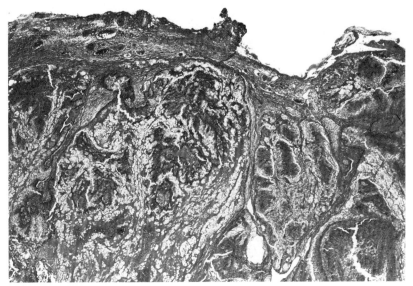

× 25

Fig. 41. Carcinoma of sebaceous glands

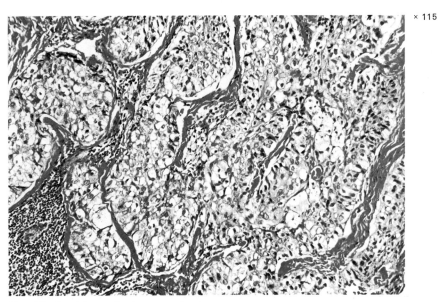

× 115

Fig. 42. Carcinoma of sebaceous glands
Meibomian gland

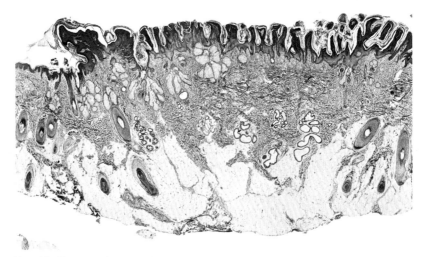

Fig. 43. Naevus sebaceus of Jadassohn

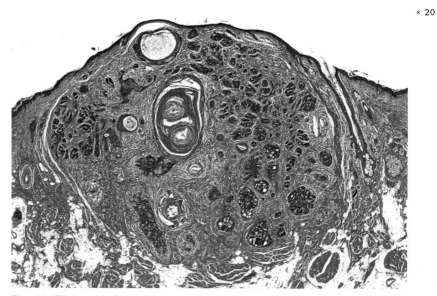

Fig. 44. Trichoepithelioma

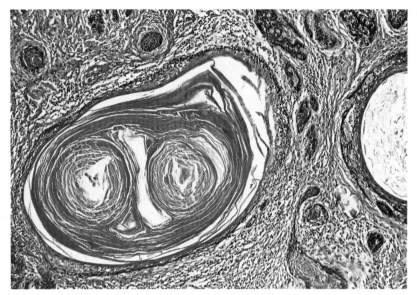

Fig. 45. Trichoepithelioma

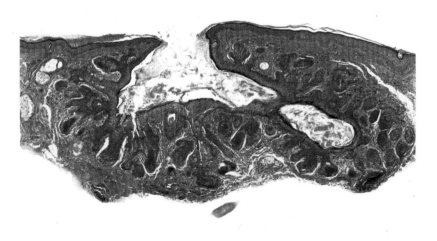

Fig. 46. Trichofolliculoma
Marginal follicular pattern

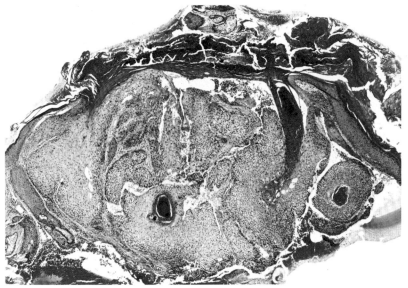

Fig. 47. Trichilemmoma
Keratin cores resemble hair shafts

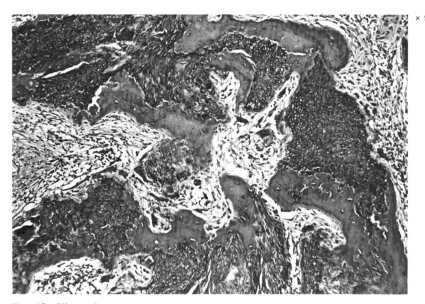

Fig. 48. Pilomatrixoma
Ossification in stroma

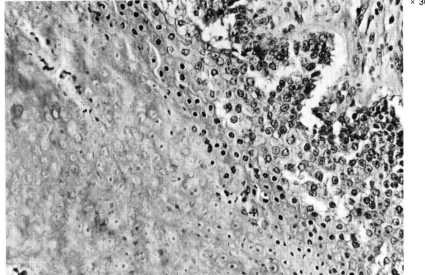

Fig. 49. Pilomatrixoma
" Ghost cells "

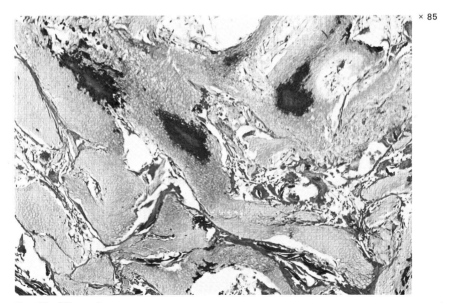

Fig. 50. Pilomatrixoma
Calcification amidst " ghost cells "

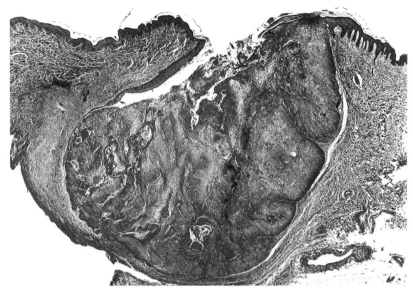

Fig. 51. Inverted follicular keratosis

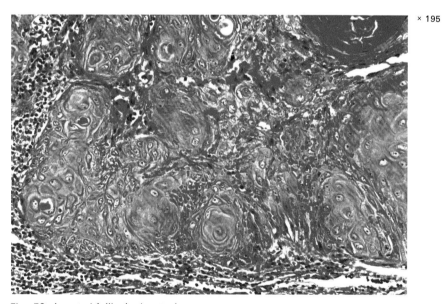

Fig. 52. Inverted follicular keratosis
Squamous eddies

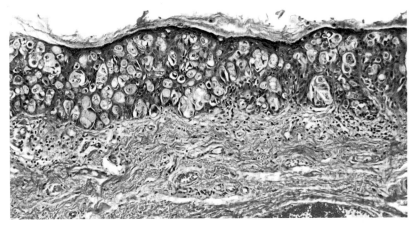

Fig. 53. Extramammary Paget's disease

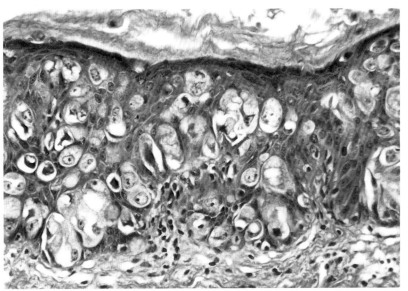

Fig. 54. Extramammary Paget's disease
Mucin cells compress epidermal cells

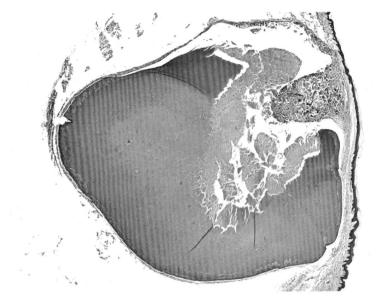

× 11

Fig. 55. Pilar cyst

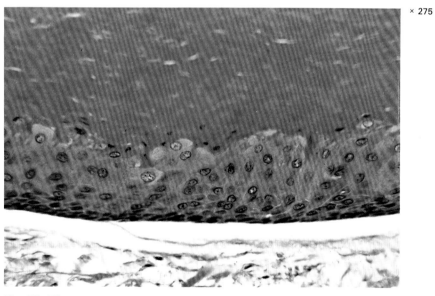

× 275

Fig. 56. Pilar cyst

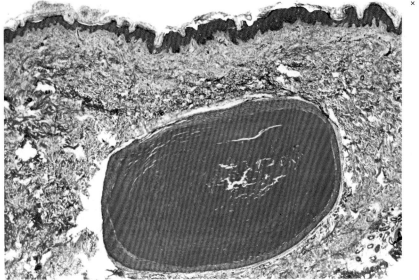

× 30

Fig. 57. Epidermal cyst

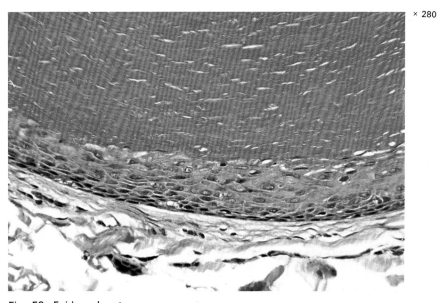

× 280

Fig. 58. Epidermal cyst

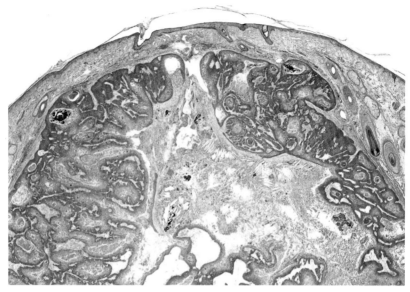

Fig. 59. Epidermal cyst
Proliferating cyst

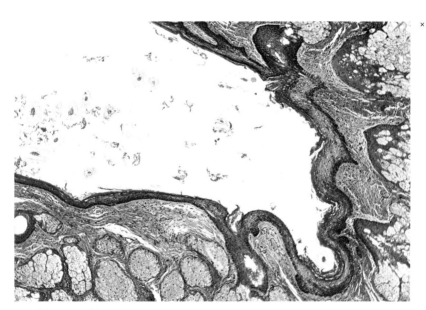

Fig. 60. Dermoid cyst
Hair follicles and sebaceous glands in wall

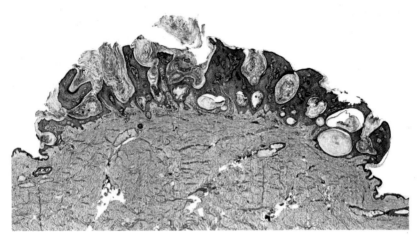

Fig. 61. Seborrhoeic keratosis

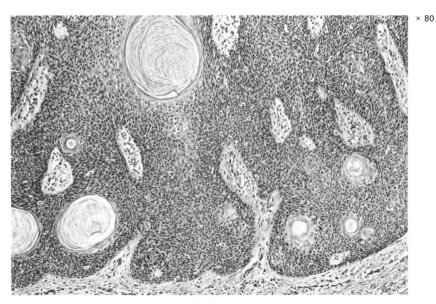

Fig. 62. Seborrhoeic keratosis
Horn cysts

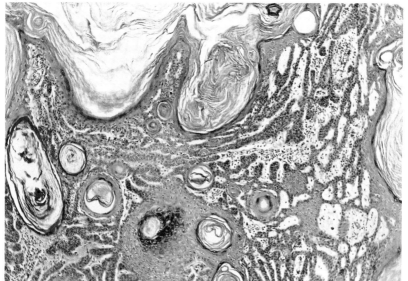

Fig. 63. Seborrhoeic keratosis
Reticulated pattern

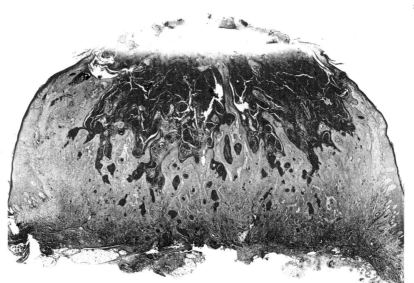

Fig. 64. Keratoacanthoma

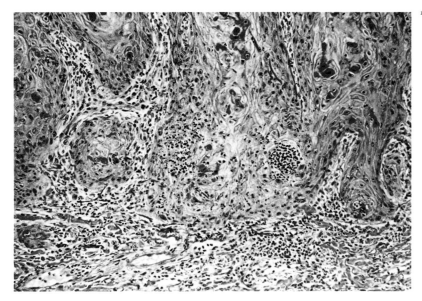

Fig. 65. Keratoacanthoma

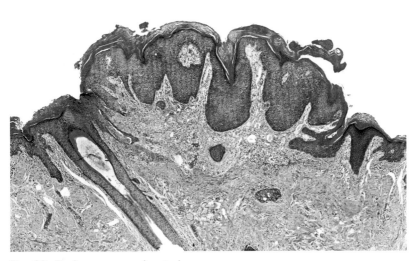

Fig. 66. Benign squamous keratosis

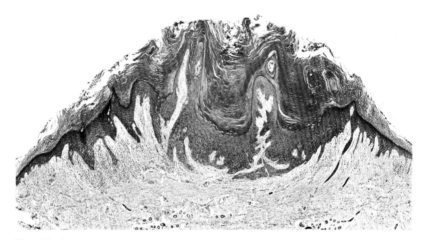

Fig. 67. Benign squamous keratosis
Note absence of basophilic degeneration of dermis

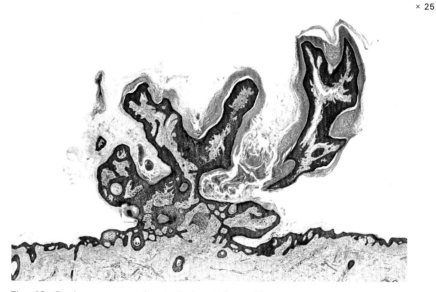

Fig. 68. Benign squamous keratosis, keratotic papilloma

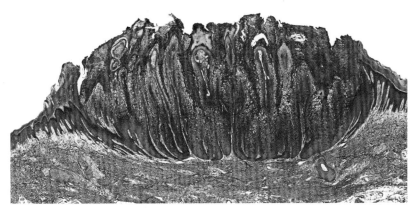

Fig. 69. Verruca vulgaris
Elongation and inward bending of rete ridges

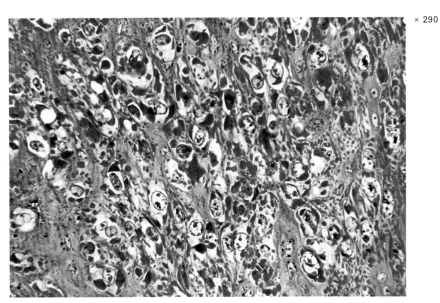

Fig. 70. Verruca vulgaris
Cytoplasmic and nuclear inclusions

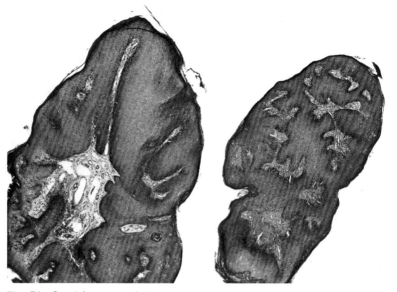

Fig. 71. Condyloma acuminatum

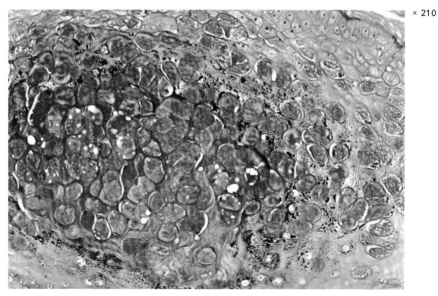

Fig. 72. Molluscum contagiosum

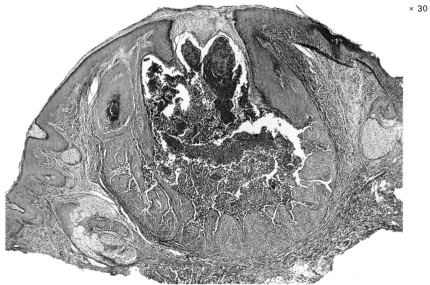

× 30

Fig. 73. Isolated dyskeratosis follicularis

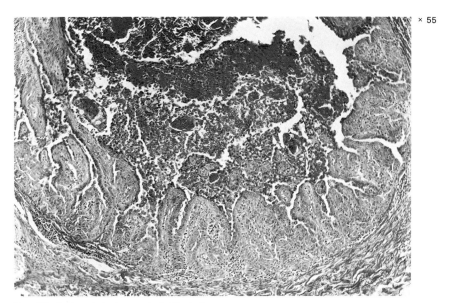

× 55

Fig. 74. Isolated dyskeratosis follicularis

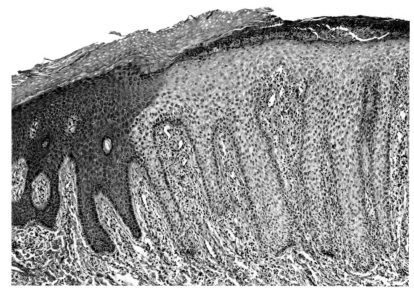

Fig. 75. Clear cell acanthoma

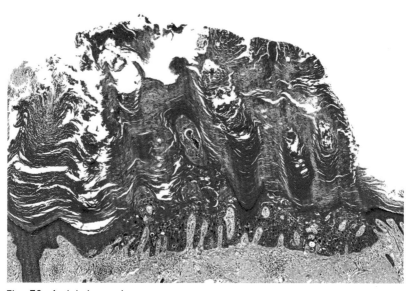

Fig. 76. Actinic keratosis
Retained horn

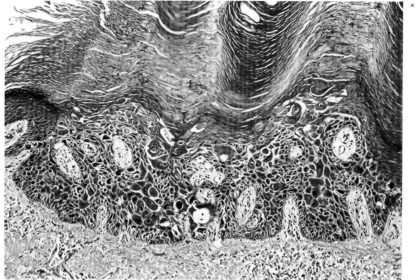

Fig. 77. Actinic keratosis
Marked dysplasia

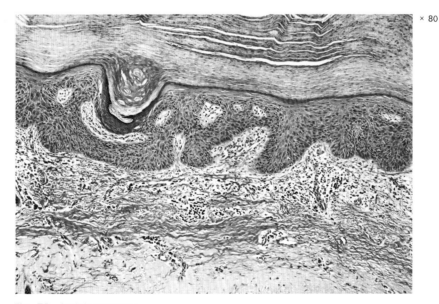

Fig. 78. Actinic keratosis
Base of cutaneous horn. Basophilic degeneration of dermis

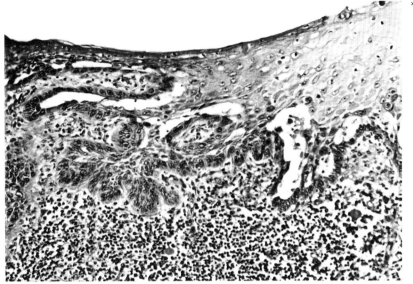

× 140

Fig. 79. Actinic keratosis
  Tubule-like extensions into dermis and clefts above basal layer

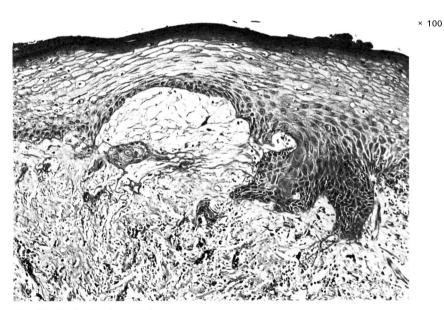

× 100

Fig. 80. Radiation dermatosis

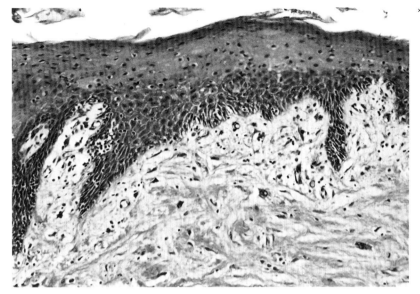

Fig. 81. Radiation dermatosis
Abnormal fibroblasts

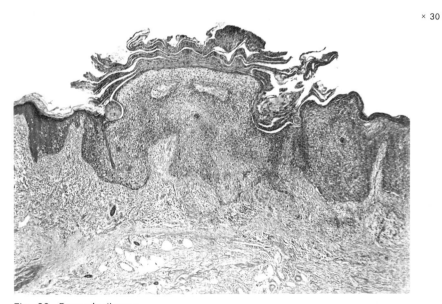

Fig. 82. Bowen's disease
Plaque-like involvement of epidermis

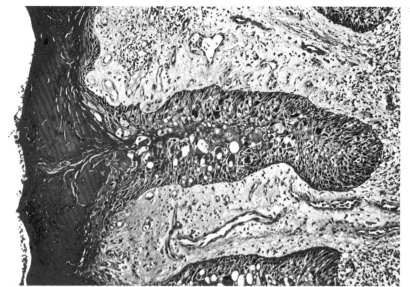

Fig. 83. Bowen's disease
Clumped nuclei

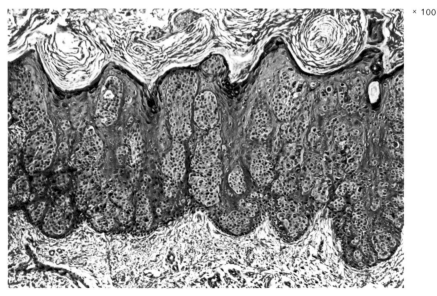

Fig. 84. Intraepidermal epithelioma of Jadassohn

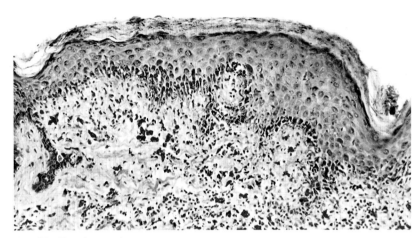

Fig. 85. Xeroderma pigmentosum

× 280

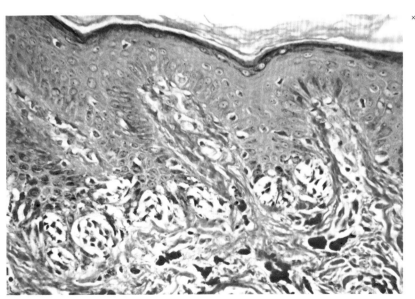

Fig. 86. Junctional naevus

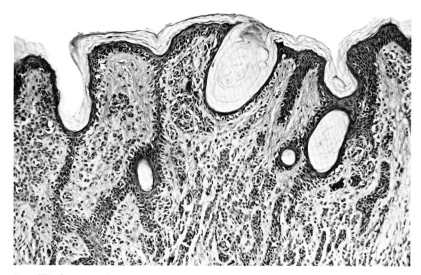

Fig. 87. Compound naevus

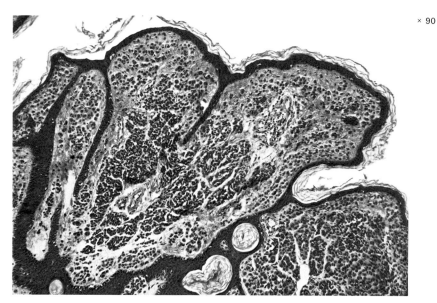

Fig. 88. Intradermal naevus

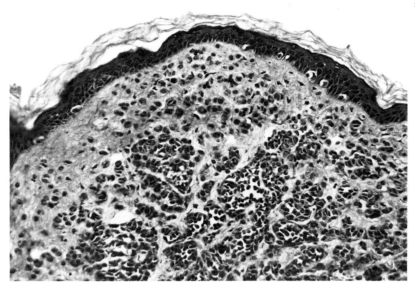

Fig. 89. Intradermal naevus

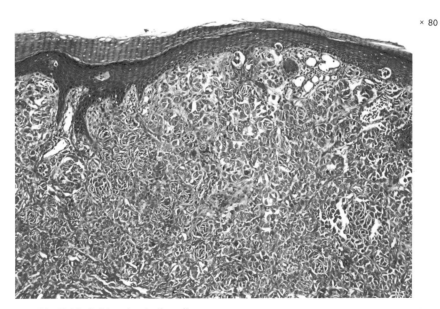

Fig. 90. Epithelioid and spindle cell naevus
Predominantly epithelioid pattern

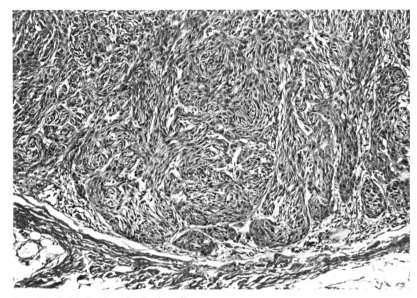

Fig. 91. Epithelioid and spindle cell naevus
Same tumour as Fig. 90. Predominantly spindle cell pattern

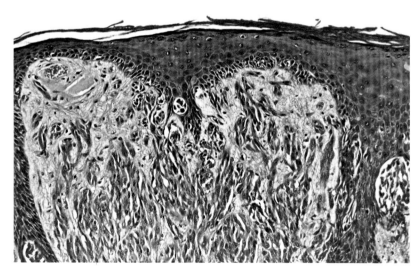

Fig. 92. Epithelioid and spindle cell naevus
Subepidermal oedema

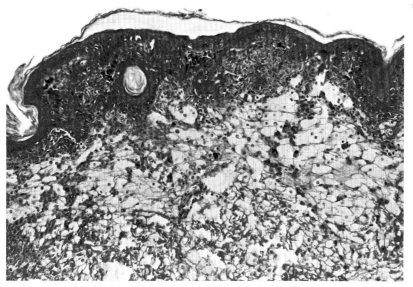

Fig. 93. Balloon cell naevus

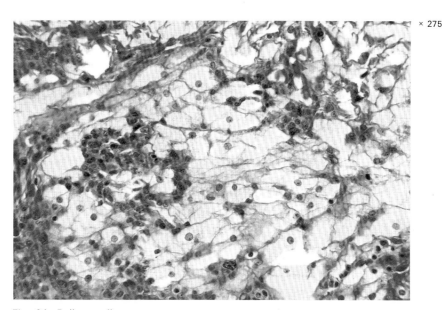

Fig. 94. Balloon cell naevus
Ballooning of naevus cells

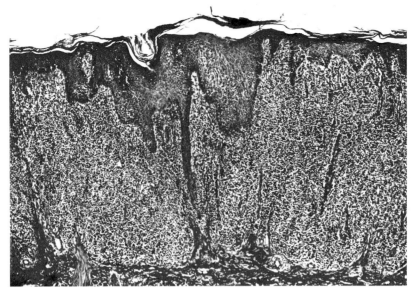

× 50

Fig. 95. Halo naevus
Dense inflammatory cell infiltrate

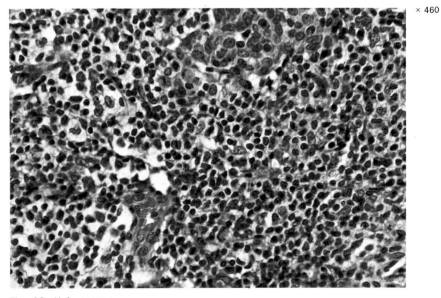

× 460

Fig. 96. Halo naevus
Dense infiltrate including histiocytic cells. Remnant of naevus cells recognizable in upper
half

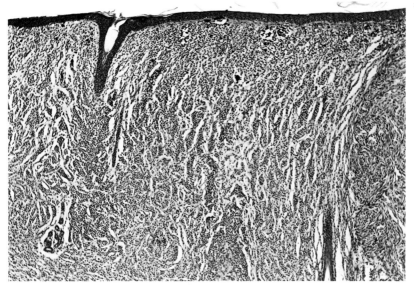

× 50

Fig. 97. Giant pigmented naevus with malignant melanoma developing on right

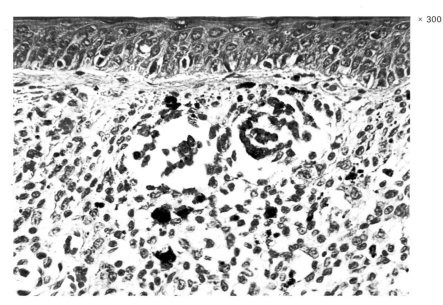

× 300

Fig. 98. Giant pigmented naevus
Naevus cells in dermis

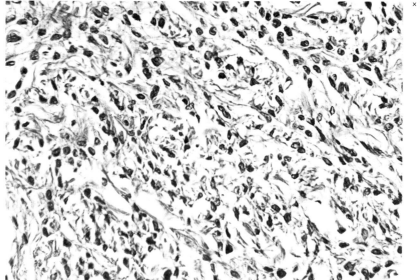

Fig. 99. Giant pigmented naevus
Loose pattern of naevus cells characteristic of base of lesion

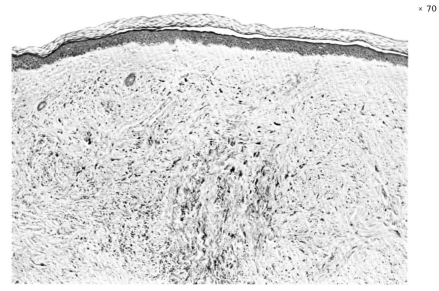

Fig. 100. Blue naevus

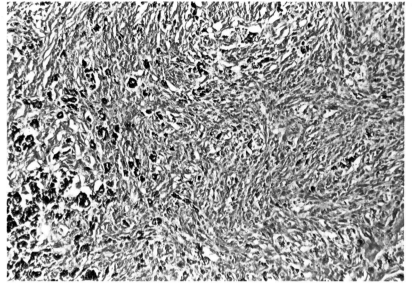

× 115

Fig. 101. Blue naevus
Markedly cellular

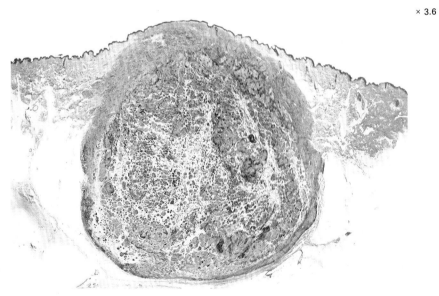

× 3.6

Fig. 102. Cellular blue naevus

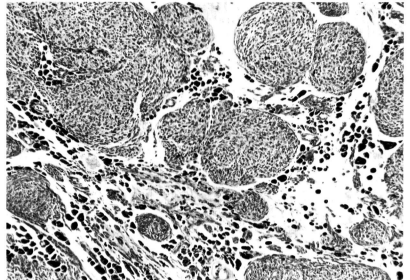

Fig. 103. Cellular blue naevus
Characteristic coils of naevus cells

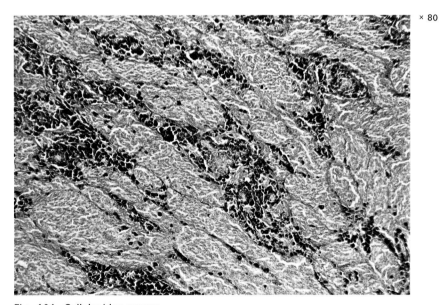

Fig. 104. Cellular blue naevus
Trabecular pattern

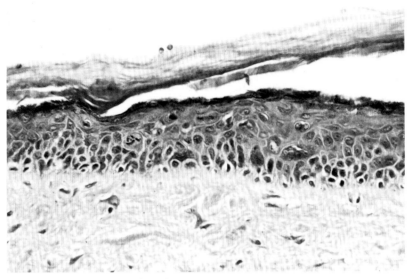

Fig. 105. Precancerous melanosis
   Early change, atypia, absence of rete ridges, mitotic figure

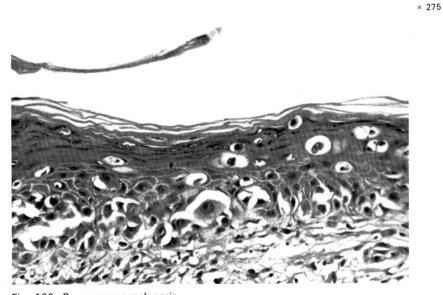

Fig. 106. Precancerous melanosis
   Atypical vacuolated cells throughout epidermis

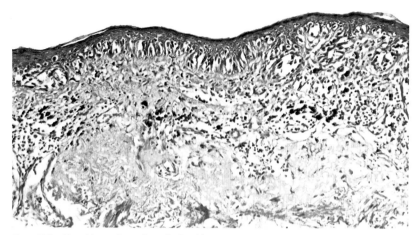

Fig. 107. Hutchinson's melanotic freckle
Face

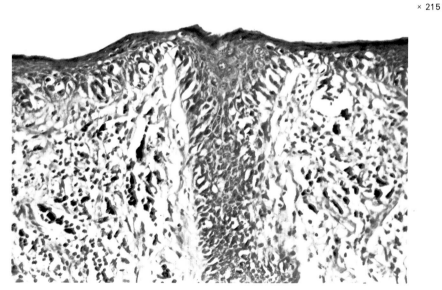

Fig. 108. Hutchinson's melanotic freckle
Involvement of hair follicle. Face

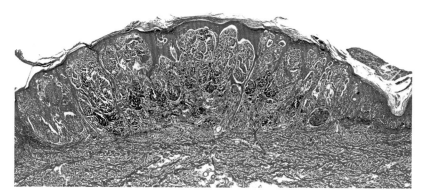

Fig. 109. Malignant melanoma

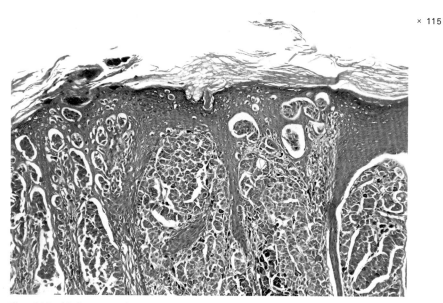

Fig. 110. Malignant melanoma
Variable pigmentation

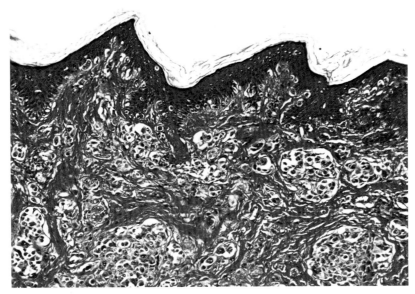

Fig. 111. Malignant melanoma
Epidermal-dermal junction. Lack of pigmentation

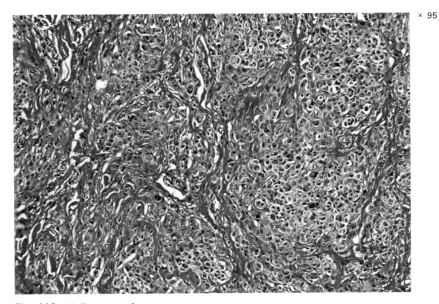

Fig. 112. Malignant melanoma
Epithelioid cell pattern. No pigment

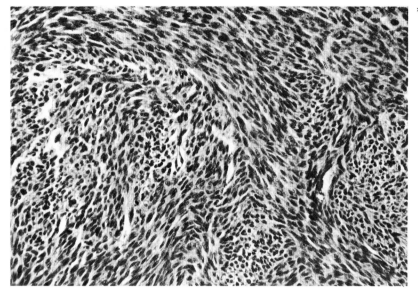

× 215

Fig. 113. Malignant melanoma
Spindle cell pattern. Little pigment

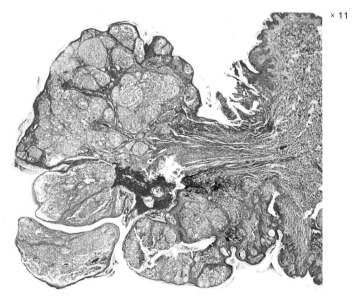

× 11

Fig. 114. Malignant melanoma
Pedunculated tumour

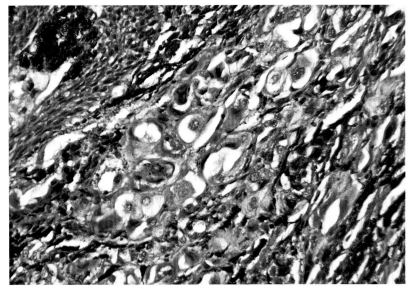

Fig. 115. Malignant melanoma
   High magnification of pigmented area in stalk of tumour in figure 114

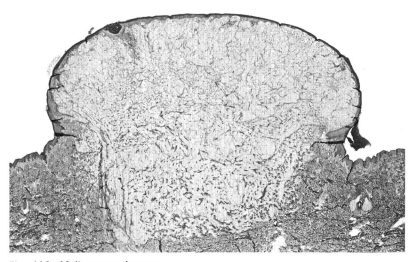

Fig. 116. Malignant melanoma
   Balloon cell pattern

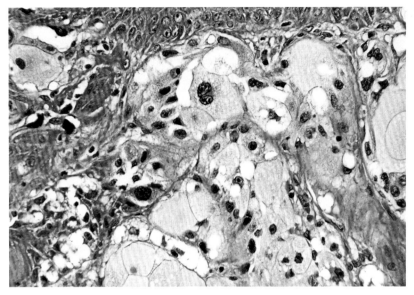

× 275

Fig. 117. Malignant melanoma
Balloon cell pattern. Same tumour as figure 116
Tumour metastasized to regional lymph node

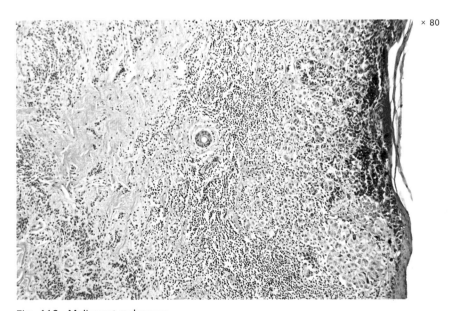

× 80

Fig. 118. Malignant melanoma
Partial regression. Remnant of naevus in lower dermis

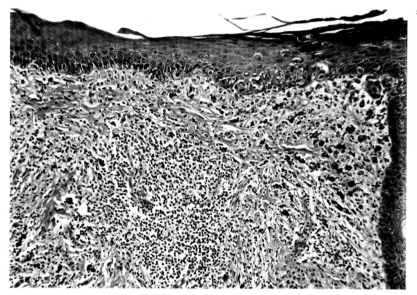

× 115

Fig. 119. Malignant melanoma
Area of regression

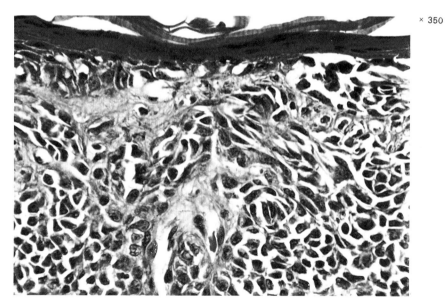

× 350

Fig. 120. Malignant melanoma arising in a melanotic freckle of Hutchinson

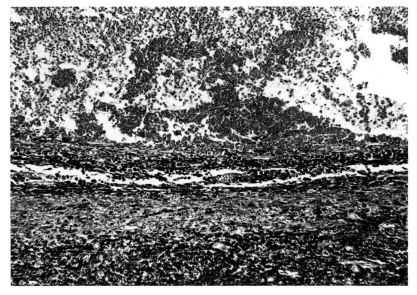

× 80

Fig. 121. Malignant melanoma arising in blue naevus

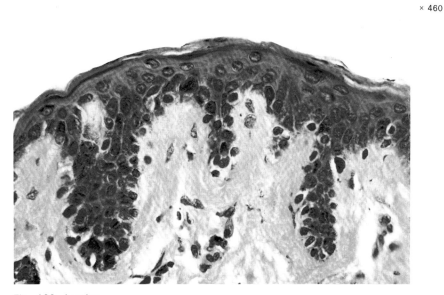

× 460

Fig. 122. Lentigo
Heavily pigmented, elongated rete ridges

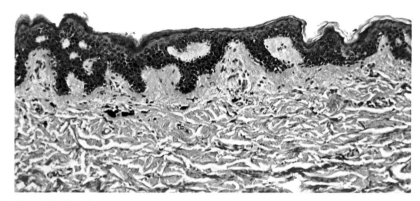

Fig. 123. Ephelis
Area of heavy pigmentation in essentially normal epidermis

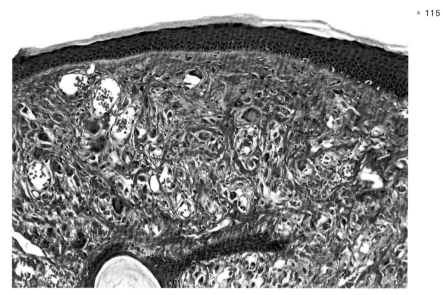

Fig. 124. Dermatofibroma
Touton giant cells

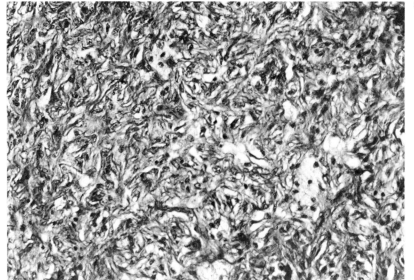

Fig. 125. Dermatofibroma

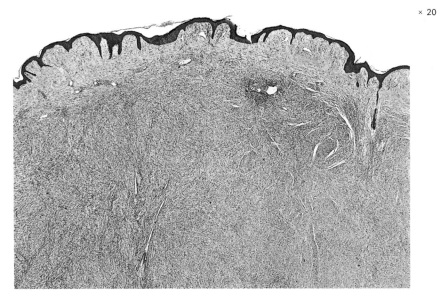

Fig. 126. Dermatofibrosarcoma protuberans

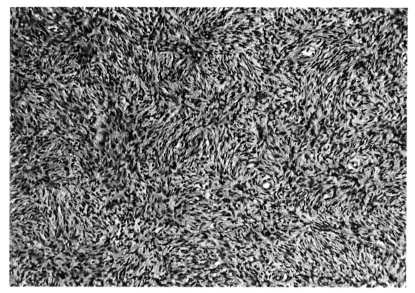

Fig. 127. Dermatofibrosarcoma protuberans
Storiform pattern

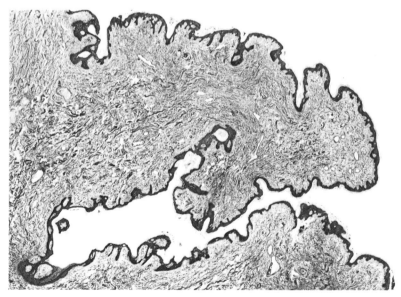

Fig. 128. Cutaneous fibrous polyp

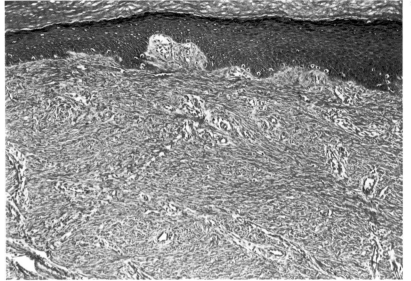

× 80

Fig. 129. Hyperplastic scar

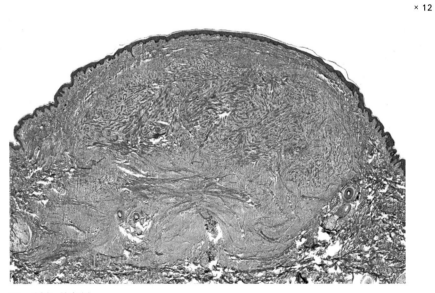

× 12

Fig. 130. Keloid

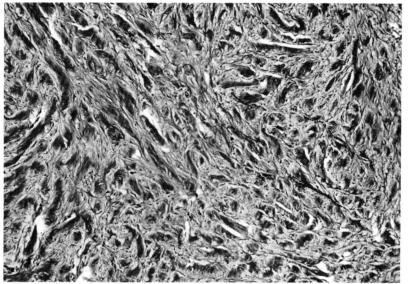

× 80

Fig. 131. Keloid
Characteristic hyaline bands

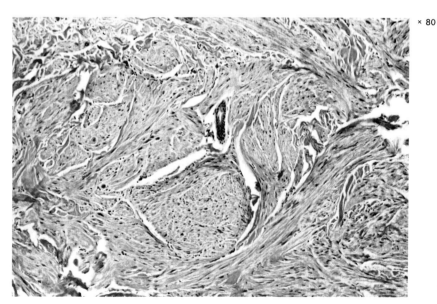

× 80

Fig. 132. Leiomyoma

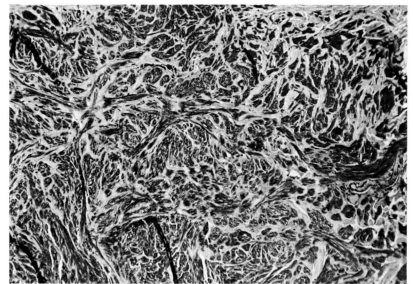

Fig. 133. Leiomyoma
Picro-Mallory stain

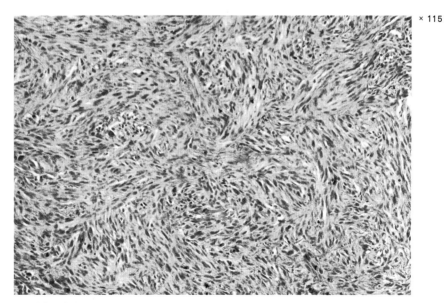

Fig. 134. Leiomyosarcoma

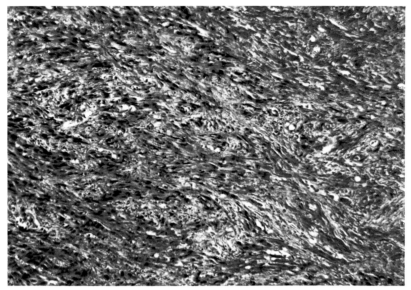

Fig. 135. Leiomyosarcoma
Masson stain

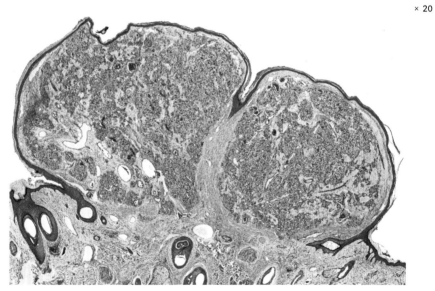

Fig. 136. Haemangioma of granulation tissue type

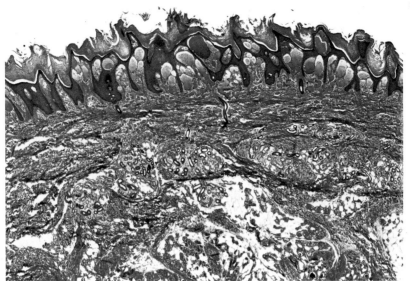

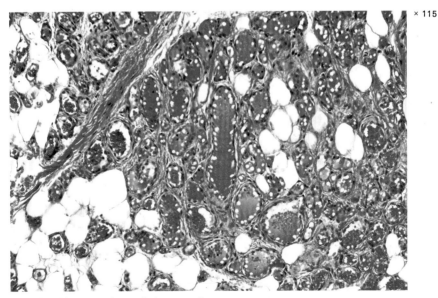

Fig. 137. Verrucous keratotic haemangioma
Angiokeratotic pattern

Fig. 138. Verrucous keratotic haemangioma
Same tumour as Fig. 137. Underlying haemangioma

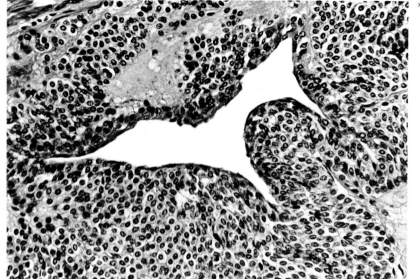

× 250

Fig. 139. Glomus tumour

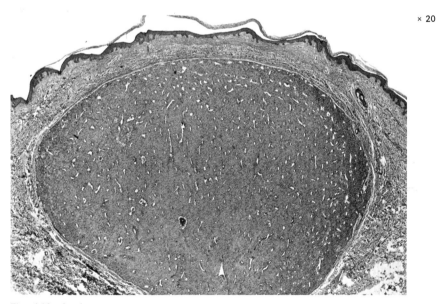

× 20

Fig. 140. Angiomyoma

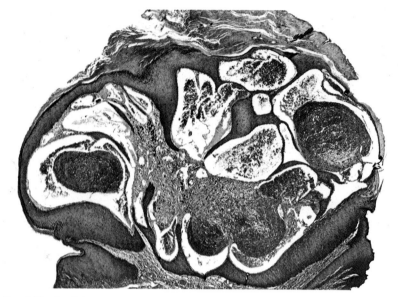

Fig. 141. Angiokeratoma
Organizing thrombi

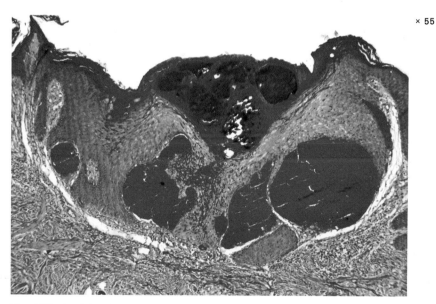

Fig. 142. Angiokeratoma
Marked acanthosis

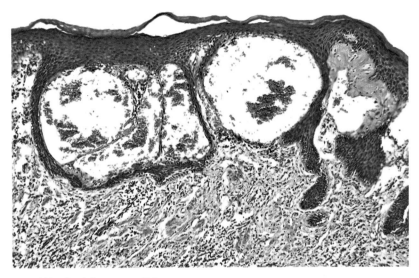

Fig. 143. Angiokeratoma, Fabry type

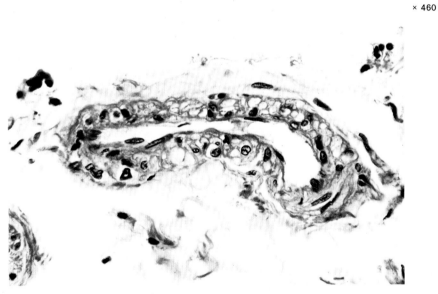

Fig. 144. Angiokeratoma, Fabry type
Vacuolated smooth muscle cells

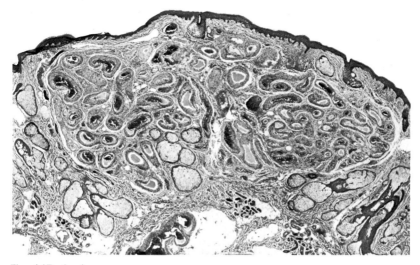

Fig. 145. Angioma

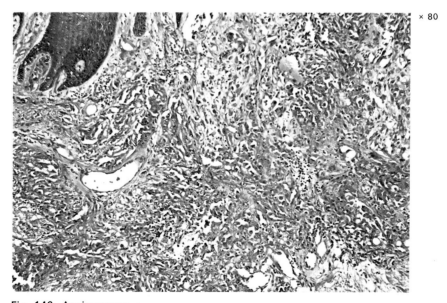

Fig. 146. Angiosarcoma

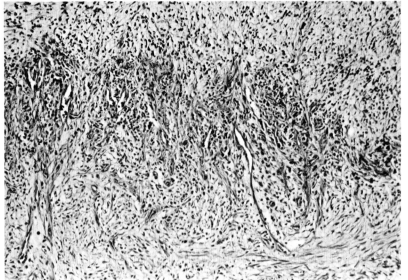

× 115

Fig. 147. Kaposi's sarcoma
Granulomatous stage

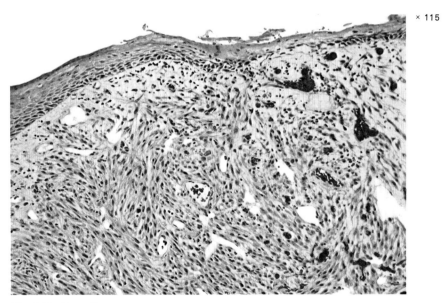

× 115

Fig. 148. Kaposi's sarcoma
Tumorous stage

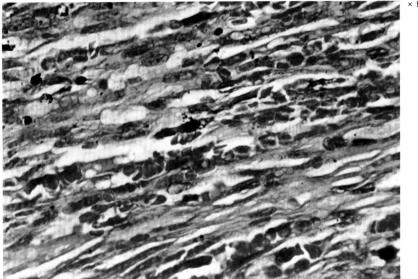

Fig. 149. Kaposi's sarcoma
Vascular slit pattern

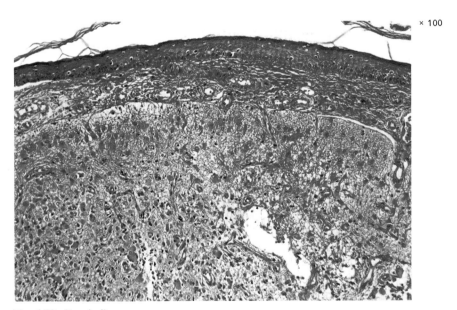

Fig. 150. Nasal glioma

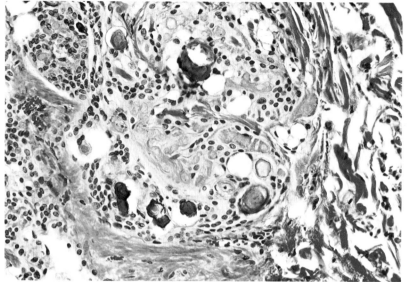

Fig. 151. Cutaneous meningioma

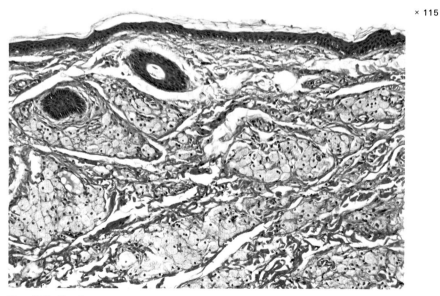

Fig. 152. Xanthoma
Eyelid

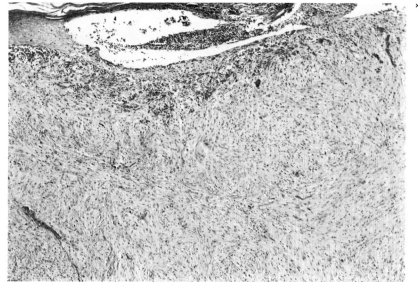

× 50

Fig. 153. Atypical fibroxanthoma

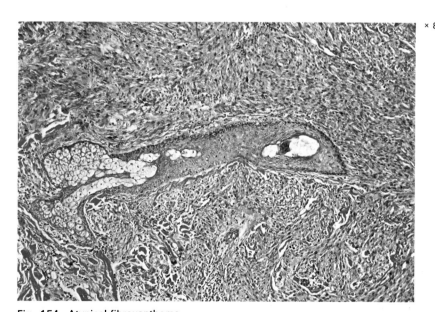

× 80

Fig. 154. Atypical fibroxanthoma
Preserved part of pilar structure

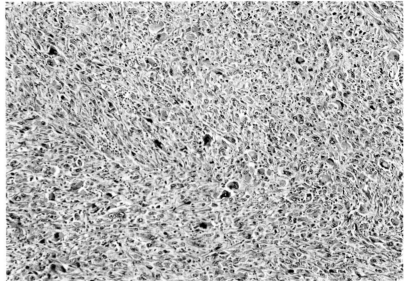

× 80

Fig. 155. Atypical fibroxanthoma
Pleomorphic cells

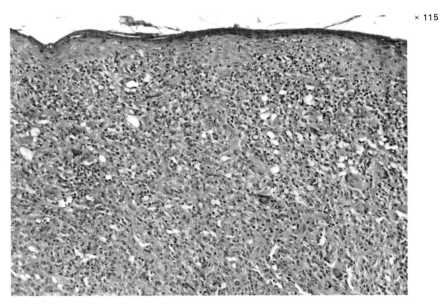

× 115

Fig. 156. Juvenile xanthogranuloma

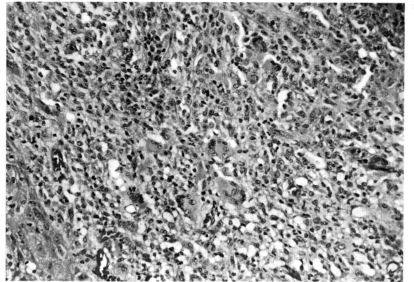

Fig. 157. Juvenile xanthogranuloma
Touton giant cells

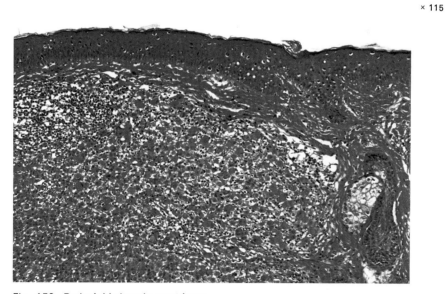

Fig. 158. Reticulohistiocytic granuloma

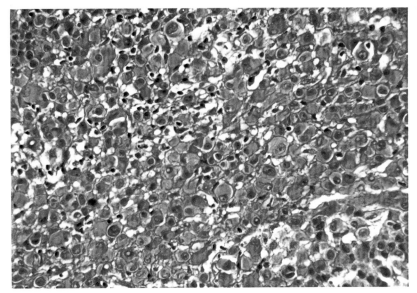

× 280

Fig. 159. Reticulohistiocytic granuloma
Large histiocytes

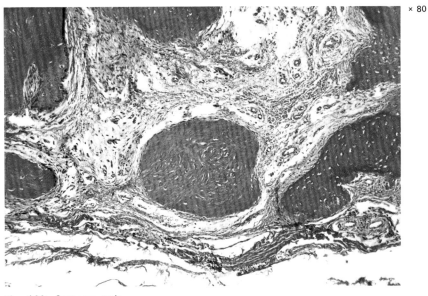

× 80

Fig. 160. Osteoma cutis

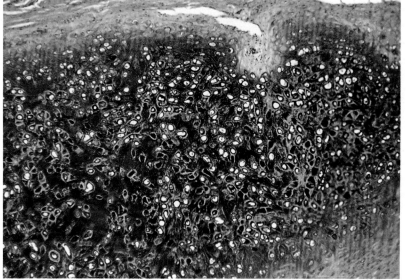

× 80

Fig. 161. Chondroma cutis

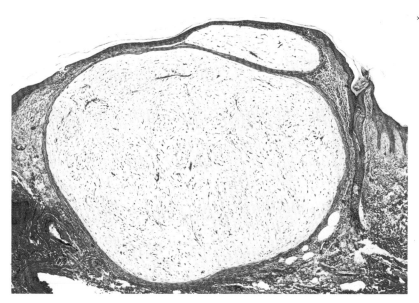

× 27

Fig. 162. Cutaneous myxoid cyst

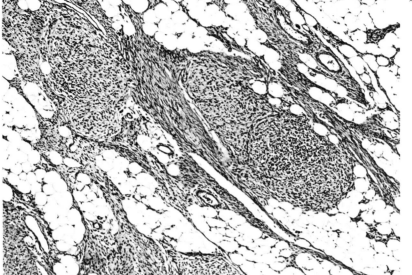

× 60

Fig. 163. Fibrous hamartoma of infancy

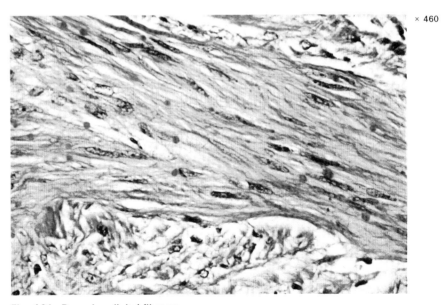

× 460

Fig. 164. Recurring digital fibroma
Eosinophilic inclusion bodies

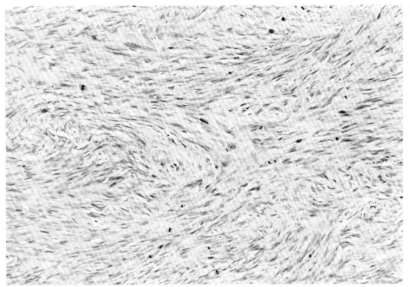

× 115

Fig. 165. Pseudosarcoma
Numerous mitotic figures. Similarity with leiomyosarcoma

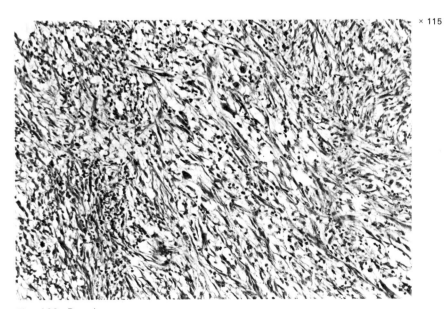

× 115

Fig. 166. Pseudosarcoma
Similarity with nodular fasciitis

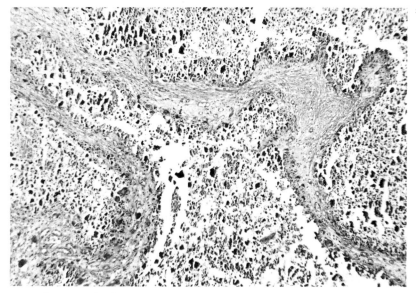

× 50

Fig. 167. Tumoral calcinosis

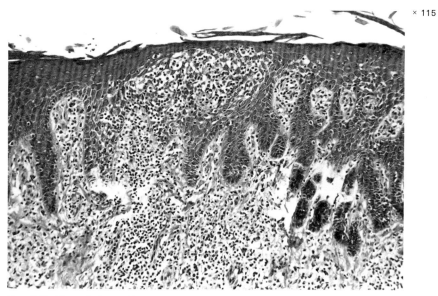

× 115

Fig. 168. Mycosis fungoides
Infiltrate breaking up part of epidermis

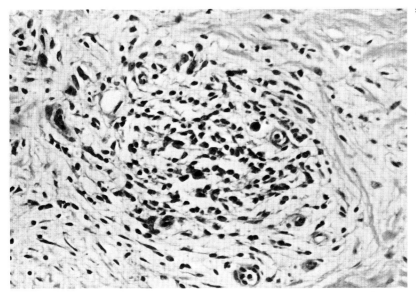

× 280

Fig. 169. Mycosis fungoides
Polymorphous infiltrate

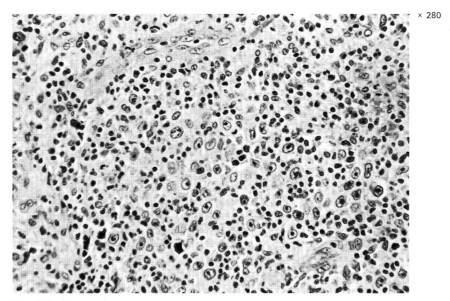

× 280

Fig. 170. Mycosis fungoides
Transition to reticulosarcoma

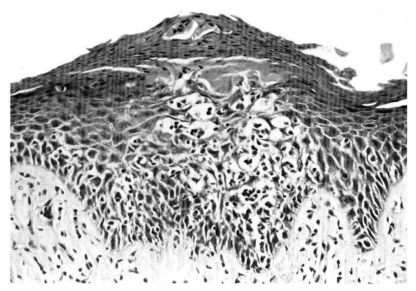

Fig. 171. Mycosis fungoides
Pautrier " microabscess "

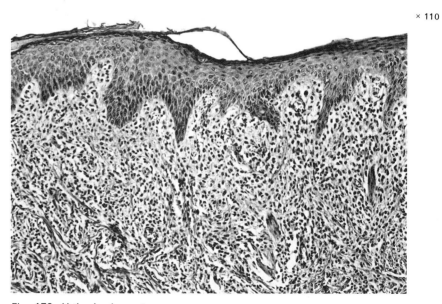

Fig. 172. Urticaria pigmentosa

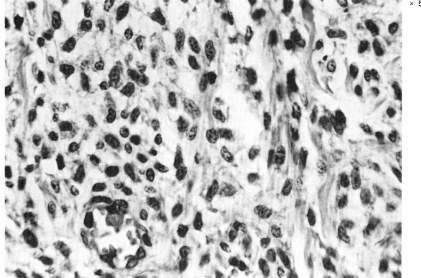

Fig. 173. Urticaria pigmentosa

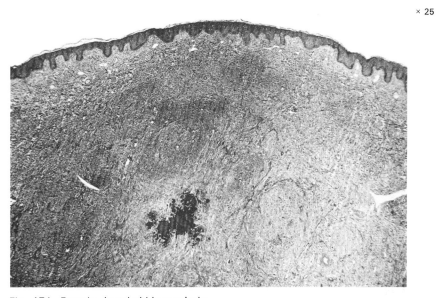

Fig. 174. Reactive lymphoid hyperplasia
1-year-old tick bite. Calcified remnant of proboscis

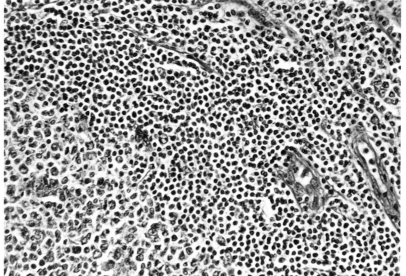

Fig. 175. Reactive lymphoid hyperplasia
Same case as Fig. 174

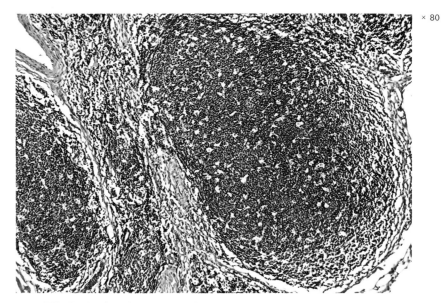

Fig. 176. Benign lymphocytoma cutis
Lymphoid follicle formation. Histiocytes present